# Intermittent Fasting Diet Guide

*A Complete Step-By-Step Guide for Heal Your Body, Weight Loss, Fat Burn and Live in a Healthy and Happy Way with the Autophagy Process (Meal Plan with 60 Recipes).*

## Jennifer Cook

# Table Of Contents

# Introduction

Losing weight, getting in shape and a healthy lifestyle is all what we need nowadays. Many people out there are looking for the best options that can help them to be in a good shape and manage weight. In order to achieve the required results, people are using a number of tricks and following tips. In the weight management industry, though, there is a number of trends coming up for anyone who wants to have the best shape and body type.

If you want to lose weight the very first thing that comes on your list is diet, of course; it is known that you need to cut down your food intake. Some people strongly believe in this trick while others do not. Some fitness freaks believe in taking food of good quality and doing exercise properly. They claim that with proper workout and exertion you will be able to cut down the fats and reduce weight.

In general, both claims are good enough. As a matter of fact, these tricks and tips work amazingly for people who persistently used them. However, in some scenarios, all these methods do have some reactions on people: for instance, some are not good enough with workout and weights, so they may collapse. Differently, others opt some hardcore dieting that cause them to lack some of the essential minerals in the body.

To be in good shape and follow a healthy pattern it is necessary to employ some of the safe and recommended solutions. Only diet or exercise are not acceptable, so it is necessary to combine them with methods that actually work. Exercise never refers to hitting the gym; if you are doing any physical activity, it means that you have an exercise arrangement in your routine. Moreover, dieting never asks you not to eat, but to eat properly.

Other than these methods, there is the fasting method. This approach helps you to make a major difference in your overall appearance and fitness plan. All you need is to ensure what kind of fasting you are going to start. Here in this book, it is written everything about the intermittent fasting: its types, tricks and diet options. It is a complete package for you to get started today and observe your results.

# Chapter 1
## Intermittent Fasting

On your way to a healthy and balanced life with a well-toned body, you came across with so many options. If you want to go for something that will help you in a long run without damaging health, then intermittent fasting can be the choice. It is something that keeps your lifestyle balanced: it surely helps you to avoid taking the heavy and junk food options and it makes you sure to digest everything you eat.

Commonly, we put on weight because the food we ingest is not digesting perfectly. When our food is perfectly digested, we will be able to make a visible change in ourselves. Fasting is one of the helpful ways to make you digest food properly in a balanced manner, in order to have the best nutrients from food. It will not let the fats and energy stored in the body as well; in fact, all the contents of our diet are digested and utilized correctly in our body.

## What Is Fasting?

Before getting into the intermittent fasting, it is necessary to understand the concept of it. Most of the people relate it to starving and keeping the stomach empty for long hours. It is a considerable fact that fasting is not just about keeping the stomach empty or starves for no reason. In some part of the world people fast as a religious obligation while, some of them, use it as a method to be in shape and lose weight.

Studies show that to achieve the better health standard, it is necessary for a person to keep the stomach empty for about 10 to 12 hours. It helps a person to make the use of all the body fats and ensure the complete utilization of the energy. Generally, we are unable to hit the empty stomach because we take the meals after intervals. In these intervals, our food is not able to digest and burn properly in the body.

However, with fasting things change and they are quite different. When a person fasts for almost 12 hours, it burns the stored fuel inside; this helps to reach an empty stomach and some extra fuel used from the reserves. Overall, it is helpful to have a balanced and attractive body.

### *Systematic procedure*

It is a notable fact that fasting is not a random act that one can do on his/her own. A systematic procedure needs to be design according to a pattern. The use of patterns helps a person to hit the right results. In case, if you do a random fasting, you will face the consequences, not the result for the effort. So, make sure you are going to have enough knowledge about the fasting, its techniques and other important details.

**What Is Intermittent Fasting?**

Intermittent fasting is becoming a trendy way to lose weight. It is considered the best way to slim down in short time. Besides that, it is also improving metabolic health and even extending the lifespan. The most amazing part of intermittent fasting is that it has a few methods. You can opt the one that suits you.

Losing weight is not an issue now. You just need to make up your mind and need some courage. Select any method from the intermittent fasting methods, as all the approaches are effective and they will give you promising results.

Intermittent fasting is an eating schedule: it alternates eating and fasting. You set a period of eating according to your goal and after setting the eating time, you have to stick to it. Remember to eat only during eating hours and fast for the rest of the hours.

In the past, it was used to treat people suffering from obesity, diabetes, and epilepsy. Now it is used to lose weight and it is a healthy method that helps your body to function in a better way.

## Intermittent Fasting And Weight Loss

We have discussed that intermittent fasting have been used for multiple purposes: it has been a treatment for some health problems and issues that includes diabetes, epilepsy and even obesity. Intermittent fasting is one of the ancient and known method that helped a number of people to slim down and get a healthy lifestyle.

While you are looking into the weight loss journey from the point of intermittent fasting, the procedure is quite clear and normal; there is no science involved in it. The only thing that comes in, is the schedule and a complete routine chart so, once a person is doing it right, he/she will get the best results.

## How Intermittent Fasting Helps To Lose Weight?

Usually, in weight loss and management, the professionals do not recommend to starve your body; they have methods to help you increase your metabolism and manage the overall diet to ensure the best outcomes. However, in case of intermittent fasting, things are quite different and advanced: the professionals suggest you to try the fasting in order to get rid of extra fats from the body. The fasting is not random but a systematic procedure that eventually helps you to achieve the right size. Here is a procedure that you need to follow:

### *Start with the short intervals*

To achieve the right results from intermittent fasting, it is important to start with the short intervals. We need to make our body familiar with the feeling of fasting. It is helpful to make things easy to digest and appealing for the body as well. If you start up with the long intervals, you may not be able to get the desired results, as they will directly cause you to lose the energy levels and you will not be able to perform the daily task. Make sure that you are going to train the body first, and then will lead things to the larger limits in getting the problem sorted.

### *Never leave the stomach empty but make it empty*

Intermitting fasting is not about starving or keeping your stomach empty. In fact, it works on a better and rapid metabolism by letting the stomach to use all the food in it and consume energy from it till the end. It is possible when you take short meals and the interval between them is longer than usual. It helps the stomach to work properly and get the best energy out of the food portion that you have taken in a specific time.

### *Using the stored energy*

Through intermittent fasting, you can remove fats by using them in regular work. It is obvious that you need some energy to perform tasks. That energy comes from the food we eat or fuel we have stored in the body. When we eat something, we consume the energy that is required and the rest of it gets stored in the body, and lastly it becomes fats. To reduce weight and fats it is necessary to get rid of that stored fat from the body. In this scenario, the important thing is to breakdown fats again in the useable energy and gets them out from the body.

In the procedure of intermittent fasting, the body gets into the position to disintegrate the stored fats energy in the body and then consumes it. Although it takes time, it really works and it gets you to the easiest way out to reduce weight.

# Chapter 2
# Intermittent Fasting Benefits



The method of intermittent fasting is not popular because it is in trend. In fact, this is something exceptional that actually helps a person to clear many problems. It is not just the weight loss that is achieved from the fasting, but there are also a number of benefits that we cannot measure. For a healthy, prosperous and balanced life, it is one of the best and possibly effective strategies. This method does not focus on your body shape, but it supports the other organs and overall body structure too.

Unlike other methods of healthy living and weight loss, fasting makes you even stronger: not just about a lighter body but its purification and health that last for long. It is good to find out about the ultimate benefits of the intermittent fasting, therefore you can do it by heart and you will know what you are going to get out of it.

## How Intermittent Fasting Helps?

Most of the people question how intermittent fasting can help you to lose weight or purify the body; the answer is simple. When you have calculated intake of food with a guided chart, then you will be using the other possible and healthy options to keep the balance of your body. A systematic procedure works in specific intervals to let your body release all the toxins, and it improves the body immunity as well.

### *Purification of the body*

This process helps you to purify the body and organs as well. When we take a meal for the first 8 hours and then we fast for the next 16 hours in a day, it means that we will take the selective food only. The food should be something that takes time to digest and provides us the energy, gradually. Moreover, during the fasting timings, we will focus on the detox water, herbal tea or other electrolytes to maintain the glucose level. The selection of food will definitely exclude the fast food and energy drinks from the diet. In the end, we will be relying on the natural options like fruits, whole wheat and vegetables; it will help to boost the metabolism and reduce the overall toxins.

### Structural transformation

Fasting supports you to make some of the amazing structural transformations. It is not just about the fat reduction but to get the muscle definition and structure designing. If you want to be in a specific body shape, with the help of the intermittent fasting and workout, you can make a real difference in your appearance too. Both factors together support you to sustain a position that you always wanted to have.

### Inner cleansing

For a healthy and presentable personality, we mainly focus on the outer cleansing that starts from the apparels to the skin. However, to sustain the personality you should have inner cleansing that purifies your organs and keeps your blood clean as well. Intermittent fasting plays an integral role in cleansing your body from inside that leaves and impact on every cell and its formation too. From the blood cells to the tissues and even organs, it makes everything clean and purified in your body. However, this purification is directly linked with your routine and the food intake you are having in the period. Make sure that you are not going to compromise the routine and you are following the best diet plan for the intermittent fasting. It will make you get the desired results in the end.

### Healthy organs

Due to our poor diet management and lifestyle, we commonly face a number of health issues and problems. Kidney stone, liver issues, diabetes, heart problems, hypertension, and so on. All these issues are related to the poor performing organs in our body. These organs are mostly under threat, due to careless diet plans and poor weight management as well. With the support of intermittent fasting, we can make our organs healthy and take care of the essentials that keep up running in our life. Studies evaluate that people following healthy diet with intermittent fasting, have organs with better health and do not face much health related issues. In fact, it helps them to recover any damage happened to the organs by keeping the things in control and scheduled.

### *Better immune system*

Most of the problems that come up to our body is due to weak immune system; it increases the chances of infections and bacterial attacks. Intermittent fasting is not just limited to the weight control or organ purification. In fact, it is linked with the overall immune system and body balance.

### Health Benefits

It is not possible to evaluate and record the health benefits of intermittent fasting. Intermittent fasting has a number of benefits that cover up multiple dimensions, so we cannot conclude any specific benefits. However, it overall makes you feel healthy and cover up some of the critical health issues for you. Here are some direct benefits that you can get from the intermittent fasting.

### *Treating diabetes*

People suffering from the diabetes can use this method to keep their glucose level in blood controlled and avoid any other issues. For them it is important to take care of what they eat and how they eat. Everything is related to total consumption and its reaction to the people. With the help of intermittent fasting, a diabetic can actually enhance the overall immunity levels and make visible changes in the diabetic conditions.

### *Rescue Alzheimer*

We all are afraid of losing anything, no matter if are money, things or even memories; we do not want to take risk with anything. Nonetheless, Alzheimer is one of the diseases that takes gradually all the memories from our brain away. It is not a sudden problem but with the passage of time it causes trouble in cognition, coordination and retention of the information as well. Intermittent fasting is one of the solutions to help a person with Alzheimer, as long as it enables the body and mind to fight against the disorder and secure the memories from being completely lost.

### *Fat and weight reduction*

Another major benefit that has made the intermittent fasting popular is the weight and fat reduction from the body. The logic is simple, when you are taking limited meals for a specific time, you consequently are taking limited calories. However, all your activities are on the same page, so you are consuming more calories than your intake; finally, it will put a direct effect on your body, weight and fat layers.

## Better metabolism

When you are not overloading your stomach with a lot of food and giving it time to work properly in time to digest it, then you are working to improve your metabolism. Eventually the stomach will be able to digest and process food properly; this will help you to get all the nutrients absorbed properly in blood and take all the benefits from it. Moreover, it will encourage you to avoid any kind of stomach problems, as your food is completely digested.

## Clean blood flow

During the fasting hours, as per schedule you need to take water, electrolytes and herbal teas that help you to clean up blood. The more we drink water, the more we detox, to finally get the blood purified. Moreover, it increases the blood flow to the whole body and in every organ as well. The better blood flow helps all the cells to receive the oxygenated blood and makes them healthy. Overall, you will get the best body health from the inside out. As a matter of fact, better blood flow helps the skin to breath, it makes it tighten and bright as well; therefore, you will not only get a good body shape but radiant skin too.

### *Proper organ functioning*

Once you have better blood circulation to all the organs, providing them nutrient, proper rest, and exercises, it means that your overall health is getting better. It will make these organs function properly and you will get the best of lifestyle.

### *Reduce stress*

Other than the body health benefits, this approach helps you to get rid of the psychological problems as well. The ultimate diet plan with a balanced exercise can help you to deal with the psychological stress problems. Good food and healthy lifestyle make you feel relax and let out all the negativity that reduces stress and makes your life peaceful.

## Intermittent Fasting & Obesity

Intermittent fasting and obesity have a strong connection to each other: it is one of the appropriate solutions for all obese people. The fasting offers you multiple strategies to maintain and manage diet plans and meal intake. This ultimate range gives you the benefits of selection, as per preferences and adjustment. The meal strategy helps you to ensure the ultimate treatment to your obesity and it also helps you to manage it.

### The ultimate solution

If a person selects the diet plans to reduce weight, then cravings are the worst enemy of that person. Getting stick to a strict diet plan is a hard choice for anyone. A person needs to cheat and have some other relaxation as well. On the other hand, hitting the gym is not possible for everyone. There are issues with strength, timings and dedication as well. Therefore, a person is left with the intermittent fasting; it is the only solution that lets a person to eat what he/she likes, works out a little and loses weight in real numbers. With fasting, you can take the meal in the meal hours and the rest is your fasting time, so you will have time to consume the energy you have taken in the meal.

### Long-term results

Intermittent fasting is not like the other options of diet plans or gym. Any skip from these options will cost you much and you will get back to the previous shape. Instead, it lets you to have the long-term results. You will not put the weight on back until you are not careless about your regular intake. Moreover, it will become your routine that you will love to prolong.

### Easy going and routine procedure

Following this meal plan approach and skipping is not a difficult task. You have the option to decide the calorie intake and you can shift from one strategy to the others. It overall helps you to maintain a cycle and stick to the lifestyle; it will not bother you much or you will not strive to quit it as soon as possible.

### No side effects

Intermittent fasting has no side effects, unless you are not taking things for granted. A few things need to be considered for sure. You are not supposed to skip the meals for more than 16 hours. If you are skipping the meal for long, you need to take the calories in other meals accordingly, so you will not be drained. You need to take the electrolytes, exercise and water along with some fruits in your fast timings to keep the energy level in the body. Overall, if you are following a good schedule there is no side effect on your side.

### Time is the key element

If you think that with intermittent fasting you will be able to feel the results quickly, then you are wrong. Expecting the magical results within no time is the issue. Commonly we become unsettled, when it comes to follow the results. In the intermittent fasting time is the key element that costs you. We do not put on weight within day, it takes weeks and months. The same thing happens when we are trying to dissolve fats and reduce weight; it will take months and sometimes year as well to get the visible results. It is important to consider that you need to keep practicing the routine without any break and you will get the results in time.

### Know the body differences

The body type of every person is not the same. Some people have soft fats that are dissolved easily in less time, while others have hard fats that take time. Therefore, you need to know the body difference in the first place, so you can have the right results; this helps you to make your strategy accordingly and will take things forward as well. All you need is to determine your body type and except results as per your case. Do not fall into the trap of someone else's experience, as they are different from you.

# Chapter 3
## Who Can Do Fasting?

We know a lot about the intermittent fasting and we can understand that it is one of the ultimate solutions to many problems. However, we need to understand that it is a limited-edition solution that is available for some specific people. We cannot generalize the application or adaptation of the intermittent fasting, as it can have multiple effects.

Intermittent fasting is all about managing your meals and whole day activities. The need for meal for a day activity can be different from one person to another, one age to another and even in genders. In this regard, it is necessary to identify whether a person is eligible for intermittent fasting or not. Things can be tricky but it is not hard to evaluate whether you need to look into it or not. Here is a schedule where is explained who can do intermittent fasting or not.

**Guide For Kids**

There is no doubt that intermittent fasting is one of the efficient tools in weight management and obesity control.

However, there is not enough evidence available to make it safe for the kids in their growing age. Kids and adolescents are in their growing age and they need the best of nutrients; they have a routine that involves physical exertion, learning new things and consuming energy, so they need to have regular meals, snacks and even some healthy options in their meal plan. Intermittent fasting can cause a barrier in the nutritional acquisition of these kids; therefore, to give them a healthy and balance life it is necessary to focus on their diet in the growing age.

The studies show that it is not a good idea to put your kid on intermittent fasting in his growing age. If the child is obese or need some weight or diet management, then many other options to help the child are available. Other than intermittent fasting, you can follow these tips:

### Plan all the meals

There is the best way to plan up the meals for your kids: you need to keep the meal time and snack time specifically adjusted, so the kids will get everything on time; moreover, you need to manage the portion for everything, in order to get the balanced nutrients.

### Purify the intake

The energy drinks, sugar beverages, cold drinks, excessive sweets, processed foods and junk foods cause obesity in kids as well. You need to purify their intake to the maximum and incorporate fresh fruits, vegetables and all healthy food items to their meal plan. Doing so, it will help them to get all the natural minerals and grow solid.

## *Promote mindful eating*

Most of the kids lack at the mindful eating: it is about when the kid is eating with intention and attention. It is not good to force a kid to have a meal when  is not mindful eating, or when he/she is playing game or watching TV with his/her meal. The kid should focus on the food and he/she should enjoy every bite of it. The strategy can help the kid to fell the taste and get full after the meal.

## *Mealtime is family time*

Make sure to serve your kids a meal with family: they should sit together with the family and eat properly. It encourages them to finish their food with concentration and it will develop a sense of discipline to them.

## Intermittent Fasting And Women

Intermittent fasting for men and women has a different approach. It is not necessary that both genders have different effects of the meal plans and fasting. For women it is important to consider whether the plan is suitable for them or not. There can be multiple reactions they could face for to intermittent fasting. The routine we develop do have a direct effect and impact on our hormonal balance, moods and psychological cognition as well.

Females are commonly considered as sensitive people, when it comes to react against the hormonal or diet changes. Therefore, for women it is necessary to assess their potential, in the first place, and then pick up the right meal plan for them.

### Ideal plans for women

We cannot rationalize the meal plan and ideas for men and women in the intermittent fasting. Both have different needs, demands and reaction to the things. Thus, it is important to pay attention to their needs and possible reaction when designing a meal plan. Here we have some ideal plans for women that can help them to get the quick and fruitful results from the intermittent fasting. These plans come with a minimum risk of reaction or problems for female. The plans are designed according to the needs, reactions and body types of female in general.

### Eat – stop – eat

A 24 hours protocol incorporates food intake two times a day with an interval of 14 to 16 hours in a cycle of 24 hours. For women, it is recommended twice a week and not more than that.

### *Crescendo method*

It includes the fasting for about 12 to 16 hours for 2 or 3 nonconsecutive days in a week. It is important to spread the weeks evenly across the week.

### *5:2 diets*

It is all about to restrict your calories to 25% for 2 days in a week and these can be two consecutive or nonconsecutive days as well. The rest of the days is normal to intake calories.

You can select any of the plans from the above-mentioned resources. However, all you need is to care about whether the plan suits you or not. It is important to find out whether you are comfortable with this meal plan or not. To try out what is appropriate for you, you can have the trial for short time and, if it suits you, then you can take the plan further, otherwise try another one.

### *Pregnancy is a no intermittent fasting zone*

During pregnancy, women are restricted to try intermittent fasting. In the reproduction, state female needs to have multi nutrients and a complete supply of food and minerals that help in the fetus development. In case of fasting, the mother can lose some of the integral nutrients and the overall consequences can be destructive and complicated.

During pregnancy and even after pregnancy, all along nursing, women should not try the intermittent fasting because it could cause them and the baby some of the health challenges.

However, they will put on some weight and, to keep themselves active and fatigue free, they need to try some physical workout, in order to avoid any muscle cramp or other issues.

In fact, after pregnancy and nursing, women could decide to undertake the intermittent fasting to help them to get back to shape and to avoid any health issue; even in this case they need to be conscious about what and when they are eating.

### *Different effects of intermittent fasting*

Women can face different effects of intermittent fasting. It is not just limited to women, but every human being can face different reactions of fating in general. For females, their situation is a little tricky, due to the sudden hormonal changes or imbalances: there may be occur other changes in a female body that makes the body sensitive to calorie restriction.

Some of them may feel different in their hormonal cycle, while others face the change in menstrual cycle. Moreover, it can lead to the mood swings and cramps at times. Female's body is sensitive to changes, so in some cases a woman could suffer from cognition problems or low blood sugar. In this regard, the ultimate safe side is the selection of right meal plan: women need to ensure that they will choose an arrangement that suits their body type and hormonal level as well.

*Important guidelines*

For all women who want to get start with intermittent fasting they need to focus on the following guidelines:

- Consider your meal intake preferences
- Select a meal plan for intermittent fasting that suits your casual routine
- Do not shift to the intermittent fasting meal plan instantly
- Take the small intervals in the beginning and then increase your fasting span
- Make sure to have a test run of your selected meal plan to avoid issues
- Observe any of your hormonal changes, menstrual cycle changes or mood swings
- Do not try intermittent fasting if you want to conceive, to be pregnant or nursing a new born
- Always make sure to eat healthy in your meals to meet up the nutrient requirements in the body

## Fasting And Diabetics

This diet is ideal to control diabetes; it is one of the popular and well-known benefits of the intermittent fasting. However, there is a fine line between the categories of diabetes. Commonly, people confuse the type of diabetes that can be treated with the help of intermittent fasting with the one that is incurable. There is no doubt that people can overcome their diabetes that is not supported by medicine; if a person is taking insulin and other diabetic medicines, then it is not possible to treat it completely with the intermittent fasting.

### Know your type

If you are suffering from diabetes and you want to control it using the intermittent fasting, then make sure you are going to identify the diabetic type. Once you have the idea about the type, consequently you could decide whether intermittent fasting is for you or not. People who have issues with their blood sugar level and they are in a pre-diabetic stage, they may look for an appropriate solution in the intermittent fasting.

In case of severe diabetes where patient takes insulin to sustain sugar level, he/she should not do the intermittent fasting. In such conditions, the person can face critical issues such as:

- Low levels of blood sugar
- Unconsciousness
- Life threatening situations
- Loss of control and coordination
- Intolerance to meal plans
- Drop in blood pressure and more
- Make a careful selection

For all the diabetic patients it is necessary to make a careful selection with their meal plan and intermittent fasting. It is not impossible for them to try out the intermittent fasting, but they need to pick up a suitable strategy. They cannot opt for a regular strategy, but they can take one day or alternative strategies as well.

## Bottom Line

It is not necessary that intermittent fasting is good enough for everyone. Everyone has specific body requirements and everyone should treat their body accordingly. In order to get the right and maximum benefits of a specific method it is important to use it right. For the kids and the elder who are unable to sustain without food, fasting is not an ideal option. Anyone who wants to control the body weight and mass should look for alternative approaches, instead of risking your own life.

Before starting up with the intermittent fasting, you always have the option to select the meal plan after trying it out. Make sure to gather the whole information about the meal plan and to select the right options for you, then you can make a real difference in the overall situation. In case of any problem with your fasting plan, you can always quit the plan and look for the medical help if needed.

# Chapter 4
# Intermittent Fasting With Keto Diet

When you are focusing on the intermittent fasting for weight loss, then you get to know about something else that is even magical. The keto diet follows the ketosis process to reduce the body fats and makes you lose weight. Combining both can simply trigger the results and get you the maximum benefits; if you want to have the quick results, then make sure that these are the best options for you. All you need is to incorporate both methods together and follow the plans keenly.

You can list out all the keto recipes for the meal times in your intermittent fasting, and you can take the keto meal, according to the plan. Doing so, you will get the double results from the both ends. On the one hand the intermittent fasting will help you to improve digestion and metabolism, on the other hand, keto diet will help to burn fats from the body and bring an amazing transformation.

## Keto Diet & Its Health Benefits

Keto diet is a diet combination that comes with no carbs or fiber, but high fats in food. The meal plans in ketosis are based on all fats that increase the fat burning producer in the muscles. Eventually, it helps to lose weight and get lean muscles that consequently help to mark the ultimate body transformation.

Keto diet is not just a method to reduce weight but it comes with a combination of multiple benefits: just as if the intermittent fasting gives health benefits that are good enough to give you a healthy and well-balanced life style.

### *Weight reduction*

One of the core outcomes of the keto diet is the weight reduction. Although it is a high, fats diet with no fiber and carbs, it burns body fats and let the person to be in good shape.

### *Healthy skin*

This diet is not only effective for the weight loss and fat burning but also for healthy skin: it helps to increase the blood flow and make the skin looks attractive, radiant and beautiful.

### *Improve liver health*

Commonly, we have issues with the blood purification that is due to poor functioning of liver. Keto diet helps the liver to work properly and reduces the fatty liver from the body;

furthermore, it gives better quality of blood and its circulation in the body.

### Reduced risk of diabetes type 2

The studies explain that, with the adoption of this diet, people suffering or diagnosed with type 2 diabetes got better coverage of blood sugar levels, because it helps them to control the blood sugar in their body that reduces the chances of critical condition and medications as well.

### Improved heart health

Keto diet decreases the chances of cholesterol and health problems while on the other hand it increases heart life: the proper blood circulation and better arteries are the reason behind improved heart health.

### Better brain functioning

If you have a well-planned keto diet plan, you will be able to improve the brain functioning. The more you will feel better and fresh, the better it will be for you to understand and to process the information.

### Improved PCOS conditions

In women, PCOS is one of the common and problematic medical conditions, as it causes a number of factors such as infertility, change of hormones, obesity, and many others. With the help of ketogenic diet, women are able to control all the negative impacts of the PCOS. In fact, they can have the improved health situation that will help them to deal with the complications easily.

## Do's & Don'ts In Keto Diet

Overall keto diet is generally safe for everyone but in exceptional cases, such as elders, kids, pregnant women and others, there is a need of consideration. Just like the other methods, it is necessary to make sure that you are not going to make any random decision about following keto diet and intermittent fasting together. There are certain do's and don'ts of the keto diet that you should know before jumping into it. These guidelines can help you make the best out of what you are going to do, so make sure to go through the guidelines keenly.

### *What you should do in keto diet?*

There is something that comes favorable when you are following a keto diet and some things are acceptable. In your acceptable things, you will get the option to use a product but not in abundance. Here are some things that you can include in the meal plan:

### *Fats and proteins*

In your keto meal plan, you need to have all the meal designs and adjusted in a high ratio or proteins and fats. The more fats you will have in the meal, the best it will be for you. Make sure you are going to pick up the animal fat and protein, instead of any artificial source of proteins.

## Portion everything

It is ideal to have the portion of multiple things in your plate. As you cannot get much rice and bread, you need to add on some portions to the food in order to will help you to get the belly filled.

## Provide yourself variations

Meat, eggs and cheese can be boring for you in a long run. You need to find out some other variations for your meal plan, so it is necessary for you to evaluate what can be the different on the menu. There are a lot of keto recipes out there, so you can pick up any of these attractive and interesting recipes. These will help you to make a real difference in your overall diet routine.

## Plan all the meals in detail

The time for keto diet plan varies from a person to person: there is not any boundary for the time that you will get results in a specific standard. Things can be different for you and to others as well. As a matter of fact, all you need to do is to design the plan for first 3 months initially; this will help you to identify how your body reacts to it. Later on, you can continue the plan for further time.

Make sure to plan all the meals separately. It includes that you will have a whole schedule for different breakfast, lunch or dinner options with you. It will help you to stick to the diet and have better results. On the other hand, multiple options in food will help you to get the different kinds of nutrients.

### Use of dairy products

Using the abundance of all dairy products is not an ideal option in keto diet. You may find the use of cheese and butter in abundance in all the keto recipes, due to high fats. Differently, you need to take only Greek yoghurt as a snack; the limit for the yoghurt is one cup or one and a half cup, not more than that.

### Things to avoid in keto diet

Just like any other diet plan, keto diet comes with some limitations and restrictions. Ketosis is a chemical procedure that happens to your body due to the high protein and fat food you take in routine. If you are not taking the food as per guided pattern, then you will not be able to hit the right results. Here are some things you need to avoid when following a keto diet plan:

### No alcohol

The use of alcohol could cause you trouble with the keto diet, as it can put effect on your stomach and eventually reduces your psychological hold. Any imbalance with the brain can cause your body to react differently and the stomach can lead to adverse reactions.

### *Avoid sugar*

Any sugar item, especially the artificial sugar, is one of the restrictions in the keto diet plan. Sugar intake increases your blood sugar level instantly and it is not a good sign, as you will not be able to consume the energy and it will not help you to reduce weight. Furthermore, you need to quit all the sweet food other than the natural sweets like fruits.

### *Limit the carbs*

Keto diet is a no carb diet. You need to avoid everything that contains carbs; it is a kind of hard thing to do and it causes you keto flu as well, because our body is not good enough sometimes to adjust. However, with a little try, you can get used to it and things will be in your favor.

### *Avoid starch in abundance*

In your keto meal plans, there is not space for the starch food products like potato, sweet potato, rice and more. It is not a hard and fat rule to cut off these products, but limit them to use; you can avoid the maximum use and occasionally incorporate these options in your diet.

## Keto Diet With Intermittent Fasting & Weight Loss

It seems to be a perfect combination if you plan to mix up the intermittent fasting with keto diet meal plans. It is not a difficult issue, as it will give you some quick results. At one side, you will have a fat cutting diet plan that will help you to reduce the body fats naturally by melting them off. On the other hand, the fasting period will help you so that the keto diet works efficiently. It is one of a system that can work for you in a long run. You can pick up the combination for quick and long-term results. Moreover, both methods do have their own benefits, so you will be able to get both of these in one package.

### *Some points to consider:*

If you have plans to start keto meal and intermittent fasting together, then you need to focus on the following points:

- Plan your diet according to your exertion and regular meal requirements
- Select a moderate fasting plan in the beginning and then take it to the next level
- Always have a trial for both in separate or combination and then make your final call
- Do not repeat the same meals but incorporate some new things to excite your taste buds
- In case of any side effect or reaction of the routine, make sure to take an exit
- You need to practice things initially and then go smoothly with everything ahead

# Chapter 5
# Metabolic Autophagy

The word autophagy is derived from two Greek words "auto" and "phagein"; these two words mean "self" and "eating".

It is a body mechanism to break down all the machinery of old cells. In the list of these old cells proteins, organelles, and cell membranes are included.  When you have no energy in your body because of less eating, this mechanism helps you to have sustain energy by regulating the cells, by recycling and deteriorating the components of cells.

You fast for a short time and eat healthy food in autophagy. Healthy food contains low carbs and high fats. It is a simple and easy way to lose weight and gain health benefits.

**How Does Autophagy Work?**

It works be keeping in the maintenance mode. It perfectly activates in the situation of stress, and its objective is to protect your body, helping you to slow down your aging process. It boosts the natural ability to perform your body's functions. It also reduces the chances of different diseases by reducing inflammation.

### *Intermittent fasting:*

While doing autophagy it is better to do intermittent fasting; you should choose the 16:8 fasting, which is the best option. With this option, you fast for 16 hours and eat in the remaining 8 hours; be careful, you cannot ignore its importance in losing weight and keeping you fit.

### *Metabolic autophagy:*

Your body's metabolism has two sub-sections or categories: the first is anabolism and the second is catabolism. Anabolism is used to build in your body new physical matters, while the catabolism is used to break down the molecules. Thanks to this, you get the energy that helps in the digestion of food.

Therefore, metabolic autophagy means to maintain a balance between anabolism and catabolism, as it has an effective impact on your body and it expands your lifespan as well. By combining these two, this method helps to replaced or construct all the damaged portions of cells by bringing back the cells after constructing them in the energy steam.

With this, in real words, your body eats itself. On the other hand, it helps you to maintain homeostasis.

### Benefits of autophagy

Autophagy is a process that cleans your body's damaged cells and harmful toxins and it supports you to generate new and healthy cells. Furthermore, it also trains your body to eat itself.

It became really popular because of its advantages, apart from losing weight, it has other positive impacts too that keep your life healthy.

The most salient features or benefits of autophagy are discussed here.

### Metabolism works better:

Autophagy's major feature is to keep your cells healthy, by replacing all the damaged cells parts and throwing away all the toxics, as your body cells help to burn your body fats. If they work properly, they will keep you healthy and fit, because it repairs or replaces the most important part of the cell, which is called mitochondria.

Mitochondria is a part of a cell that actually burns your body fat. Besides burning your body fat, it makes the ATP, which is the energetic currency of your body. Along with the other things your cells also have some toxics that build up in the cells and damaged them badly, but getting rid of these toxins you can save your cells from harm. Moreover, it helps your cell function in more appropriate and efficient way; with this, not only your body fat burns but it also helps to make protein. All these features help your metabolism works better.

### *Weight loss:*

For weight loss, the process is an amazing element. Besides getting other health benefits weight loss comes at the top of the list. Through this, your body fats burn without damaging the protein. Autophagy activates in the short fasts burning them and preserving muscle mass and proteins.

Besides that, it also reduces the insulin levels in the body, which helps to lessen the inflammation and it stops you to gain weight. Furthermore, it also helps the cells by repairing it and it assisting in burning the fats to get energy.

### *Save your life:*

Autophagy is an old mechanism that plays a vital role in preserving your life. Firstly, it works effectively when your body is stressed, starved, or infected. During these hard times, autophagy comes into action by minimizing the damage and by doing maximum repair.

With the combination of intermittent fasting, autophagy's function gives better results: both of these starve your body's glucose contagious intruder, as it helps to boost your immune system by reducing inflammation. Animals use this technique to preserve their energy and to repair their damaged cells.

In the case of the human body, its immune system is critical; however, with autophagy, your immune system fights illnesses and reduces the risks of various illnesses. All its functions have a huge impact on your overall health and it saves your life by healing and replacing the dead cells with healthy cells.

### *Maintain homeostasis:*

Because of this, you get a vibrant health. It helps you to maintain your homeostasis. Homeostasis is a function that balances your body cells, due to this function, your body's dead cells are removed and it forms new cells.

### *Improve your quality of life:*

When we talk about anti-aging term it is not only related to your skin beauty. Anti-aging is a deeper term that goes deeper from your skin. Autophagy is an ancient method and scientists have known about this since 1950s. However, in the past it was not common but now, because of its advantages, various studies have been conducted on this process.

The last researches have shown that it is perfect for improving your cellular health by repairing them. This process does not replace the whole cell but it repairs the damaged part of the it; besides that, it also removes all the toxic elements and fixes the cells.

After the process of repairing, your cells start to work in a better and efficient way, by working like new and younger cells. You will notice that some people look younger from their actual age. On the other hand, few people seem older than their actual age and the reason behind these two conditions is the efficiency and condition of the cells. If your body has toxic and damaged cells, it will affect you in a negative way, and you will look older than your biological age. Moreover, if your damaged cells are repaired on time, it will keep you look young and fresh, so these cells play a crucial role in your appearance.

### *Improves brain health:*

Indeed, autophagy plays a vital role in improving your brain health. In many people, brain diseases develop at a later age, and the reason behind these brain diseases is the misfolded protein around and in the brain. Autophagy removes the misfolded or useless protein that automatically prevents you from different brain diseases; for instance, the disease like Parkinson and Alzheimer can be prevented or delayed.

### *Regulate inflammation:*

Regulation of inflammation is very important to save yourself from diseases because it boosts your immune system and helps you to combat diseases; furthermore, it addresses the issues that trigger the inflammation and by controlling them, it reduces the rate of inflammation.

### *Improve digestive system:*

We all know that the digestive system plays a crucial role in your life. Your life depends on your digestive system, that means: if the liver works properly, only then your body will get essential substances. The process of Autophagy helps you to improve your digestive function by removing and replacing the damaged cells, and it finally enhances the function of liver. Lastly, with the fast, your liver gets a break to reschedule its function.

The process also removes all the junk that is based on unhealthy and useless toxics or cells. By activating autophagy with a perfect schedule, it will help you. Try to expand your fast to overnight, as with this, your digestive system will get the time to heal itself.

### Protects from infectious diseases:

As autophagy strengthens your immune system, it protects you from infectious diseases, by giving you the strength to fight against them. Moreover, it eliminates certain microbes from the cell, such as HIV, Mycobacterium tuberculosis; besides, it does not only removes directly the cell part but it also removes the toxins that are created by the infections.

### Improves muscle performance:

You can improve your muscle's performance through this process. After exercise, your muscles need repair and they want energy too. Through autophagy your muscle cells will react immediately, it will improve the energy balance and will reduce the risk of damage in future.

### Minimize the apoptosis:

Autophagy plays an important role in dealing with apoptosis. This process is dangerous for cells as it caused the cell's death.

Your body generates some inflammation to clean the mess of dead cells, but it is not enough. In this situation, autophagy steps forward by selecting the cells that can't be repaired and by dumping them.

### Prevent cancer:

It also lowers the inflammation and reduces the chronic inflammations that can cause cancer. As we see, various types of cancers are increasing rapidly. One of the common cancers is breast cancer.

You will be amazed to know that with autophagy the chances of cancer reduce, as it responds quickly against chronic inflammation, DNA damage response, and genome instability; it also suppresses the process of cancer development.

### Improves your skin health:

To look beautiful, you must have good skin. You cannot get good skin by using moisturizers and other beauty products, your skin beauty also relates to your diet. An appropriate diet provides your skin nutrients.

You damage your skin cells by working in the daylight and by exposing to dust; furthermore, skin cells also are mostly affected by bacteria. Through autophagy, you can a glowing and clear skin, it also removes the damaged cells and last, but not least, it repairs the cells and removes the bacteria from the skin.

**Diet Should Follow Autophagy:**

Diet plays an important role in achieving your goals through autophagy. You must be careful about what you are eating: the first and most essential feature is to low your carbohydrates and calories intake and secondly, increase your protein intake.

### *Low-carbs food:*

The reason behind lowering the carbs in your diet is to use your body fats. Yes, your body will force to use its fats as a source of fuel. With low carbs you need to take food with high fats because proteins can turn into the carb, whereas the situation is different in the fats.

### *Protein consumption:*

You need to limit your proteins once or twice a week. Restrict protein limit to 15-25 grams. With this, your body gets the time to recycle its proteins. It reduces the inflammation and cleanses your cells; while cleaning your cells, it does not cause muscle loss. Whilst you are not taking the proteins, your body uses the proteins by consuming its toxins.

### *Diet is compulsory:*

During autophagy diet is compulsory, as you will not be able to achieve your goals without following a proper diet plan. Set the time for eating and fasting and during the eating hours don't try to eat any unhealthy food, is prohibited during autophagy.

## Metabolic Disorders & Autophagy

Metabolic disorders are affecting human life in a negative way, due to the change of lifestyle and environmental aspects. Besides, the main threat is the metabolic disorders. Autophagy is considered the best solution to avoid metabolic disorders. Indeed,  various recent studies are showing the positive effects of autophagy on human life.

### *What are the metabolic disorders?*

Metabolism is an important function of your body so that it uses this chemical process to transform the food you have eaten into the fuel or energy, and this energy keeps you alive.

When your body's metabolism process fails, then metabolic disorders emerged. Due to its failure, your body either gets less or gets much of the essential substances, and both situations are harmful to your health.

Our bodies are sensitive and cannot tolerate the error of metabolism. When your liver stops to function in a proper way, metabolic disorders occurred.

### *Common metabolic disorders:*

Metabolic disorders are complex and cause various complications. These are life taking disorders.

### Diabetes:

The most common metabolic disorder is diabetes and, unfortunately, the number of patients with diabetes is increasing rapidly.

### Gaucher's disease:

This disease occurred when a specific kind of fat doesn't break down due to the liver's inappropriate functioning.

### Hereditary hemochromatosis:

It is a condition that emerged with an excessive amount of iron in different body organs. With this metabolic disorder a man can lose his life, as it can cause liver cancer, heart disease, diabetes, and liver cirrhosis.

### What is autophagy?

According to the physiology, autophagy is known as a protective housekeeping mechanism. With its mechanism, it eliminates all the unhealthy cells and toxins. In its cellular function it aggregates the protein, constructs the damaged organelles, and invades pathogen through a dependent pathway of lysosome.

### Obesity:

Obesity is the most serious concern and a threat to a large number of populations. Due to the eating disorders and unhealthy eating people are becoming the victim of obesity. Obesity is also causing various other diseases, such as diabetes, heart diseases, and so on.

***Relationship between metabolic disorders and autophagy:***

Autophagy is protecting you from these metabolic illnesses, for instance, in obesity, autophagy plays the role of an internal source as it provides the stored nutrients during the limitation of nutrients.

As metabolic disorders can take your life you need to take preventive measures. In a few cases, there is no cure and a person can die within months, and the cause behind the metabolic disorders is the imbalance distribution of essential substances.

At this stage, the autophagy comes into action: it recycles the macromolecules and regulates the cellular homeostasis; furthermore, it cleans the damaged organelles and proteins. Recent studies showed that autophagy plays an important role in improving the human life, by preventing a person from all these metabolic disorders, or by decreasing the risks of metabolic disorders.

It repairs the cells of all the body organs and removes all the toxic and dead cells. This function enhances the function of the organs. The liver works in an effective way and it also helps with obesity and insulin resistance.

Moreover, it also eliminates all the useless amounts of the essential substance. So, it helps in balancing the cells and their functions; moreover it automatically decreases the chances of metabolic disorders.

# Chapter 6
# Intermittent Fasting 101 Methods

Here is a complete guide about the Intermittent fasting methods that are available and you can use to make a difference. These are not something unusual, but they are recommended and used methods that actually work. Commonly, people think that intermittent fasting is a kind of starving that appears to be a torture for people. In fact, it is not like that: intermittent fasting is a systematic management of the calories, food intake and its consumption as well.

Everyone has multiple options for the intermittent fasting methods. All these methods are effective and give results. Moreover, these methods make the fasting save for everyone. If you follow the right methods for the intermittent fasting, you will not starve your body; in fact, you will be providing all the necessary nutrients in the right timings.

The best thing about these methods is the management of your whole day and meal. It is not just the time but also the calorie management, so you can have the idea about what to eat and what not. You can opt the things that will help you to make a difference in the overall scenario, so make sure to select these methods carefully that are near to your potential and stamina. This will help you to get the right results from the intermittent fasting practice in a long run.

## Advantages Of Intermittent Fasting:

Intermittent fasting is really good for your health because it helps you not only in losing weight but also it looks after your health. The top benefits and positive effects of intermittent fasting are discussed here.

### *Lose weight:*

The basic reason behind intermittent fasting is losing weight; it is an effective way to lose weight, because you eat less and healthy. Moreover, it enhances your hormone's function and helps to reduce weight. With this your body fats burnt and you achieve your goal in a limited time.

### *Physical fitness:*

Besides preventing neurodegenerative disorders, it also helps you to remain fit. With intermittent fasting your metabolism works efficiently, by training your digestive system and by taking care of that you will eat in a limited time frame; it also trains you to eat only when you feel hungry. Moreover, you started to eat healthy food.

Some people believe that fasting damage your metabolism. It is totally a wrong perception. If you fast and eat in a proper way, it helps your metabolism by making it better, using fats and glucose efficiently for energy.

***Expand your life span:***

It expands your life span by improving the liver function, as you are giving a rest to your liver, and by fasting, its lifespan is extended. So, your liver becomes healthier and functions effectively.

***Prevents from Alzheimer's disease:***

As we all know, Alzheimer is a neurodegenerative disorder and it is not a curable disease; therefore, it is important to take preventive measures. A study shows that intermittent fasting reduces the chances of Alzheimer because it plays a positive role in reducing its complications by improving the symptoms.

It is also acclaimed that intermittent fasting protects from other neurodegenerative diseases too, such as Huntington and Parkinson.

## 16:8 Fasting Method

It is an easy, effective and most popular way of intermittent fasting. It is a sustained and convenient weight loss technique that also improves your health. 16:8 fasting method allows you to restrict eating time to 8 to 10 hours a day. In this method you fast for 16 hours every day and during the 8 hours of eating you can take 2 to 3 meals.

It is a simple method and you can easily do it. So, you are just skipping your breakfast. If you finish your dinner at 8 pm and do not eat anything till 12 pm the next day, you completed your fast; it means that you have just skipped your breakfast and have completed your 16 hours fast. For women, though, it is recommended to do fast for 14 to 15 hours, because for them 16 hours fasting is too much time.

You can set the cycle of 16:8 fasting; this totally depends on your preferences. So, you can do it on a regular basis, which means every day. Moreover, you can also do this twice or thrice a week. There are not any hard and fast rules like other dieting fasts, it is a flexible diet plan that can easily fit in your daily routine.

### Health benefits of 16:8 fasting:

The most important benefit of 16:8 fasting is that it attacks obesity. Yes, you can lose weight and save yourself from all the diseases related to obesity. Besides losing weight, you can also enjoy a bunch of health benefits, for example, it reduces the chances of heart diseases, cancer, inflammation, cholesterol level, and blood sugar levels, it is very effective for your mental health as well.

## *Is it right for me?*

The first question that raised in a person's mind is: is it right for me? The answer to this question is yes, 16:8 fasting is right for you. Because of this you lose your weight and it also has a positive impact on your overall health.

One thing that you should keep in mind is eating healthy food. The food must be nutritious and organic so, there is no room for processed food or food with artificial sugar. If you will not eat nutritious food, fasting will not help you at all.

## *Recommendations:*

If you have any health issues it is better to consult your doctor before fasting. For example, if you are diabetic, or have other issues, this can put you in trouble. For children, underweight individuals, pregnant girls, it is not a good choice. So, if you have any problems, don't fast without an expert's consultation because you can face serious consequences.

## What Is 20:4?

20:4 is one of the types of intermittent fasting where you fast for 20 hours and you can eat during the 4 hours. It is slightly different from warrior diet, as in this you cannot eat anything during the 20 hours of the day, while in the 4 hours you can have a big meal. It is a very common type of intermittent fasting.

It is a bit strict fasting as compared to others. In 20:4, unlike the warrior diet, you have to stick with the ketogenic diet. Yes, in warrior diet you just stuck to the low calorie's food, but in this you are supposed to eat limited items even in eating hours. You can set the eating time and fasting time according to your comfort.

### What to eat after completing the 20:4 fast?

You need to eat healthy, nutritious and ketogenic food, and it is best to start eating gradually. Unlike warrior diet, try to start eating from snacks, then gradually keep eating small portion of meals in the 4 hour-time duration. Some people eat a proper meal right after finishing the fast, and then eat snacks in the remaining time of 4 hours. The second method is okay too, but it is recommended to start with snacks.

You can eat white fish, green leafy vegetables, water, dark coffee, broth, and low carb vegetables.

### What happens during 20:4 fast?

You are not eating anything for 20 hours, but you are eating only ketogenic food in the 4 hours eating time period. This diet will put pressure on your body to use its glycogen stores that is the storage part of carbohydrates. In its reaction, your body will start burning your body fats and if you do not eat for long hours, it will lower the stay of insulin levels, so your liver will mobilize and start to use your body fats as a fuel.

## Long Fasts

Shorter time duration fast is common and is in trend. People fast for short hours to lose weight, but besides short hour fasts, you can go for a long fast, like 5:2, 16:8, 20:4 are the short duration fasts. In the list of long fasts, 24 hours, 36 hours and 48 hours fasts come. The longest intermittent fast is of a duration of 48 hours.

### *What to drink during long hours fast?*

In a long hour fasting you give yourself and your liver a full one or more than one-day break. During these two days you don't eat anything but you can drink fluids with zero-calories. You can drink water, tea, and black coffee; water is an essential fluid and if you do not drink water, your body will be dehydrated. So, drink plenty of water to keep your body hydrated during long fasts.

### *What to eat after completing a long fast?*

In shorter fasts, you can eat any healthy food in big portion; however, after completing the longest fast of intermittent fasting, you can't eat in big portion, so you need to start eating in small portions and gradually. Start your meal from light snacks and take a small portion of meal after two hours.

If you start eating instantly, it will put you in trouble because it can cause diarrhea or nausea.

### *How many times you can have a long fast in a month?*

Long hour fasts are not an easy task. Everyone cannot do this. You cannot have long fasts twice or once a week, it is strictly prohibited. So, it is suggested to have a long fast one or twice a month. As if you do it with short breaks, it can affect your health in negative way.

### *Benefits of long fast on health:*

Long fast have positive effects on your health. You put an effort and it paid off. With long fast, you find the best results: your body fats burn at a great speed and it not only helps you to lose weight, it also helps you to maintain your health.

It also plays an important role in preventing neurological disorders because it reduces the risks of cardiovascular diseases and few cancers. Moreover, it expands your lifespan and it gives you a healthy lifespan as well. Lastly, it improves your metabolism and combat inflammation that can cause various diseases.

## Fast Diet – 5:2

The fast diet 5:2 is also called the 5:2 diet. It has a symbolic name that means eating 5 days normally and limiting calories on the remaining 2 days. Here fast is a misleading term, like another intermittent fasting, you don't restrict yourself from eating for a certain time because you just limit your calorie intake. On fasting days, you just intake around 25 percent calories, as compared to normal days.

This diet was introduced by a British doctor and journalist named Michael Mosley. It is an easy effective dieting method of intermittent fasting; it does not require 16 hours fasting nor 10-hour fasting. You normally eat 5 days a week and in this method you just need to sacrifice your 2 days. Yes, only 2 days a week. You restrict yourself to 500 to 600 calories on two days of a week.

### What to eat on a fast day?

In fast diet-5:2 you can eat at any time but you need to be careful about what you are eating, because you are supposed to eat food that is rich in nutrients and it must have all the basic elements like protein and fiber.

### Vegetables:

If you start fast diet-5:2, then eat more vegetables, as it will give you a satisfaction of tummy-filling. Vegetables have low calories, so you can take more vegetables at a time, eating carrots, zucchini, and green leafy vegetables; all these vegetables are healthy and provide you enough amount of fiber.

### Eggs and whitefish:

Protein is vital while you are fasting or not, so you should eat the food with protein but with less fat. Therefore, you can take hard-boiled egg, white fish, tofu, beans, lentils, peas, and cuts of lean animal. You can use these items after boiling, roasting, or grilling; don't fry them, as it will add fats in it.

## Other food items:

Along with vegetables and protein food, you have some other options too, such as drinking water a lot. Fast days doesn't stop you from drinking water as water is vital. You can also eat fruits with less sugar, blueberries, and blackberries, for instance; soup or broth are also effective in intake during fast day.

## Patterns of eating:

You get a room while fasting 5:2. It doesn't restrict you from eating for long hours, so you can eat at any time of the day. For helping you the 2 most effective eating pattern is described here: one is three small meals and second is two slightly bigger meals.

## Three small meals:

In this eating pattern, you take a meal 3 times a day. You do breakfast, lunch, and dinner, but all these meals are small in quantity.

## Two slightly bigger meals:

You eat twice a day in this eating pattern. You skip one meal and eat medium-sized meals twice a day.

During both, the patterns must focus on nutritious food. The food must be low in calories and fats, it must be rich in protein and fiber too, and don't cross your limit of calories.

## 24 & 36 Hours Fasting

Intermittent fasting has different types of fasts that differ in duration too. 24 and 36-hour fasting are also 2 types of intermittent fasting. You can opt any one type of fasting, depending on your feasibility.

### *What is 24-hour fasting?*

24-hour fasting, as the name suggested, is a fast of 24 hours. From your last dinner to the next day's dinner you can set the time according to your comfort; it is an effective method of losing weight, as it covers more hours with fasting, in order to get the results soon. You are eating at least one meal a day.

For losing weight it is recommended to do thrice a week. For some people it is easy to fast for 24 hours. Therefore, to get the results soon they fast 5 times a week.

### *What is 36-hour fasting?*

It is a total fast of 36 long hours where you don't eat anything for consecutive 36 hours. It is an amazing way to reduce weight for even diabetic patients. Doctors recommended diabetic patients to have a 36 hour fast twice or thrice a week. With 36 hours fasting you get quicker results.

*Disclaimer:*

Fasting for 24 or 36 hours is not equally benefited for everyone. For some people, such as underweight people, ladies who are pregnant or doing breastfeeding, boys or girls under the age of 18, it is not beneficial and not recommended to fast. In addition to this, people who have eating disorders or any health challenges should not fast for 24 hours or 36 hours.

If you want to fast, then it is suggested to try it with short time duration fast. It is ideal to start fasting from 5:2 or from 16:8 fasting; if you complete those fasts, then do 24 and 36-hour fasting.

## Fasting In Alternative Days

As its name suggested, fasting in alternative days means that you fast every other day. You will find its various versions. Some believe that you need to restrict yourself to around 500 calories during a fast day, but on the non-fasting days you are allowed to eat anything; it is an effective weight-loss method. While fasting you can drink calorie-free drinks, like water, tea, and black coffee.

### An easier way to lose weight:

This fasting is also known as "every other day diet". People find it much easier as a way to lose weight, as they can stick to this comfortably, and also because you restrict your calories, rather than remain hungry for a long time. With this fasting you get the same results as you get from the other long hour fasts.

A study's results showed that fasting alternative days have various positive effects: you preserve muscle mass along with burning your body fats quickly, and if you start exercise along with the fasting alternative days, it will be a cherry on the top, because you will start to lose weight at double speed.

### *Is it safe to do fasting in alternative days?*

Studies have shown that fasting in alternative days is safer than others. It suits most of the people. One of the major benefits that you get from this fasting is amazing, as long as you don't gain the weight again. In those methods, the week you stop fasting, you start to see the changes in weight. It also decreases anxiety, depression and overeating.

## <u>Impulsive Fasting</u>

Most of the body changes we observe in ourselves are due to impulsive or mindless eating. When we are sad, we eat, when we are happy, we eat, we use to have dinners, brunches and lunches to celebrate anything. In short, for everything, we have only one way out and that is eating. Eventually, it gives us a huge feedback in the form of massive weight gain and a bad shape body as well. To fix up the problem it is important to treat it the way it needs to be.

Intermittent fasting brings you the option of impulsive fasting that brings you the pattern of fasting, similar to our food intake. As we do not think for once at least to eat anything, same as this is one of the random and rash fasting types. You adopt fasting randomly to make sure you will starve enough to let your body consume stored energy.

### Not a harsh game

Many people think that impulsive fasting is harsh one. They believe that you are torturing yourself by keeping the body starve for food in different timings. In real, it is about building your capacity to control food cravings and manage the overall metabolism. No matter it is an impulsive form of fasting, but still you need to consider the diet schedule.

### A careful selection

The most important thing with the impulsive fasting is the selection of schedule. Although there is no specific schedule for the fasting, you need to make careful selection. Fasting does not refer you to risk your life. So, make sure you are going to take the meals at appropriate time. You need to keep the fast long enough that you can handle easily.

### Not a fixed fasting chart

It is not necessary that you need to follow a fixed fasting chart in the impulsive fasting. If one day you have a meal in the morning and then after the 8 hours break, you will take another meal; then, on the second day, you may take the first meal in the afternoon. The timings are different and random, so your body will get the different treatment every time.

## Warrior Fasting

Warrior fasting was first introduced by Ori Hofmekler, who is a famous author in the field of health and fitness. He proposed this fasting in 2001, after observing its effects on himself and his friends in the Israeli special force. With this fasting, you can lose your weight in short time span.

Warrior fasting is actually based on the ancient warriors eating patterns. They used to eat less during the day and eat a lot at dinner. Hofmekler described this fasting as "it is designed to improve the way we eat, feel, perform and look".

Warrior fasting involves fasting for 20 long hours. These 20 hours include night and day time. After 20 hours you do over eating in the 4 hours duration. These 4 hours must be the evening hours.

### *Not a scientific study:*

Warrior fasting weight loss strategy is not a scientific study, but it is based on a person's observation. Thus, there is no research-based answers that are available on its effectiveness. Even Hofmekler also said that he didn't propose it after experiment; it is totally based on his observations. He observed this during his stay in the military force, so that's why he named it warrior fasting or warrior diet.

### What to eat?

There is no specific food to eat in warrior fasting, so you can take any food with healthy fats and protein. If the food is organic and nutritious you can take it. However, it is prohibited to take food that is processed or has artificial sugar.

The most common food items that you can take during the 4 hours eating break are listed here.

- Hard-boiled eggs
- Dairy products like milk, cottage cheese, yoghurt
- Grains like rice, bread, oatmeal, and so on
- Chicken or beef broth
- Fruits like mango, banana, apples, pineapples, strawberries, peach, kiwi, grapes, pomegranate, and so on
- Raw vegetables for example peas, green leafy vegetables, carrots, mushrooms, onion, and so on
- Vegetal juices of carrot, beet, celery, and so on.

### Benefits of Warrior fasting:

Warrior fasting is gaining the attention of the dietitians because of its results. Consequently, it has various benefits that help you a lot in different dimensions. A few major advantages of warrior fasting are discussed here.

***Weight loss:***

Fasting, as we all know, has a history and helps a lot in weight loss. Warrior diet is also one of the intermittent fasting types that helps you to lose weight in small duration because of 20 hours fasting you lose a certain amount of your body fats. With this you not only lose weight, but the chances of cardiovascular disease are also minimized.

***Inflammation:***

Inflammation is the leading cause of major diseases. For example, few types of cancers, heart diseases, bowel disorder, diabetes, and many others. Warrior fasting helps to fight against chronic inflammation.

***Improve blood sugar:***

Like other fasting methods, with warrior fasting, you will see improvement in your blood sugar, as it controls your blood sugar and insulin. However, it will only happen when you eat the right food during eating hours.

***Side effects of warrior fasting:***

Besides its advantages, it has many side effects too, for example, it is not an ideal weight-loss method for everyone. Some of the major side effects of warrior fasting are given below.

- Lightheadedness
- Dizziness
- Low energy

- Eating disorder
- Low blood sugar
- Hormonal imbalance
- Fainting
- Anxiety and depression
- Constipation

## Protein Sparing Modified Fasting (PSMF)

Protein sparing modified fasting, which is also known as PSMF, is a way to lose weight. This method of weight loss was launched in 1970s. and the purpose of PSMF was to help people with obesity. In the past physicians used this method, but now, due to its effective and promising results, dietitians are also using it.

### What is PSMF?

The PSMF is a diet containing low-calories and most protein. It is a weight-loss method that helps you to lose weight rapidly; in other words, "it is a diet with the goal to maintain muscle mass while losing body fats".

It is not an easy diet plan. However, it gives you great results in a short time period, as long as you take low-carbs and fats but it takes enough proteins that will preserve your lean tissue mass. Due to enough amount of protein, there are fewer chances of nutrient deficiencies.

### Phases of PSMF:

A PSMF has two phases: the first is "intensive phase" and second is "refeeding phase".

### Intensive phase:

The intensive phase of PSMF lasts for around 4-6 months. In this phase your diet contains fewer calories. The calories limit is less than 800 per day. Food like egg whites, fish, or chicken are lean protein foods but also have calories. Therefore, while eating something, you need to know what nutrition it has in store.

During this diet, you are allowed to take per day only 20-50 grams of carbohydrates. In simple words, you can take only 2 slices of bread. Considering protein intake, it varies person to person, because you need to take protein according to your body weight, like 1.2 to 1.5grams of protein per kilogram weight.

Fats are not allowed at all in the form of oils or dressings, because you are taking enough of your food.

### Refeeding phase:

The refeeding phase lasts for around 6-8 weeks. In this phase, you start to gradually increase the calories intake back to normal levels. In this, the level of carbs increased to 45 grams in the first month, while in the second month, it raised up to 90grams.

There is no certain or underline limit of calories in this phase, because it will increase naturally by the addition of fats and carbs in the diet. Food that is high in protein and fiber will become a part of your diet, so you can take any fruit or vegetable that has low-fat in this phase.

### *Is it a safe method to lose weight?*

It is very safe if you do it for a short time period and your goal is to just get a kick to start losing the weight. However, if you do it for the long-term, then you need to take some measures. For example, it is better to do it under medical supervision, because in long-duration you need to monitor various things, such as your gallstone, blood sugar levels, uric acid, and other features.

Although now we have a modified form of PSMF, it is different from the 1970s diet. Now it is more balanced and designed after research. In addition, it is suggested to do it under proper supervision.

## Bottom Line

The multiple kinds of intermittent fasting allow you to have the ultimate access to the wonderful body transformation and weight loss. It is not a random technique to be good with your health but one of the refined methods that are used anciently. Although you have so many options in intermittent fasting, you need to pick any one of these carefully, as these are similar and interlinked and mixing up the random things can cause issues or problems later.

# Chapter 7
# How To Start With Intermittent Fasting?



Intermittent fasting is getting popular among people and almost everybody is talking about this. Is this becoming a way to lose weight? To have a healthier life? Or people do it for a religious purpose?

In general, intermittent fasting is the best practice to follow a healthy and fit life for a long time. According to several researches and studies, it is noticed that the proper and restrict way to have meals with a proper schedule, not only improves metabolism, but also gives multiple other benefits as well.

Before starting the intermittent fasting it is important to know that, what it is all about?

Intermittent fasting is basically a schedule and a way to have your meals in a day. During the fasting you have to follow a pattern in which your meals are divided according to the quantity and calories necessary to take in a day, in an hour respectively. There are multiple approaches regarding the intermittent fasting meal plans and people follow the one that suits them or fulfills their requirement.

**How To Start Intermittent Fasting?**

*Choose the method*

First of all, before starting, it is necessary to identify the method that a person is going to follow throughout the fasting process. There are multiple approaches or methods usually adopted by the people during the period like:

- Sometimes people may choose the eight-hour-method where they have food or meals and rest of sixteen hours do the fasting, and in the whole fasting, is only allowed to have a non-carbonated drinks and low calorie liquid intake like water, green tea, black tea or coffee without milk and sugar.
- Some people do the fasting in alternative days like having a restricted calorie diet in a week and fast for one day or two days a week.

*Find out effects & probabilities*

When you have selected one method of fasting, then do a proper research before applying it. In other words, it is vital to consult the health consultant or nutritionist because the expert can evaluate your body type and could suggest you the best and suitable method for you. Fasting directly could affect the metabolism of a person and may do some chemical changes that could have different consequences, according to the person. Anyway, all methods are suitable an appropriate for everyone. If you put your body in an intense method, perhaps the consequences can affect you badly.

### *Know what happen to body with fasting*

With intermittent fasting the consequences are hormonal changes that take place inside the body. With the limited supply of the food and calories your body functions take place accordingly.

Fasting improve the production of hormones that are good for the muscle's growth and strength and it also helps to increase the utilization of energy that attains from the stored body fats. This will also keep the insulin level at the minimal rate, that means the body uses more stored body fats that put the body in the process of weight loss, so the body can fight more efficiently with the damage or dead cells and, finally, the body's ability to fight against disease goes high. Fasting is ultimately good for almost everyone, as well as it is an effective way to control over the weight and to follow the healthier lifestyle.

## Benefits Of Following The Fasting

In general, people only think that maybe the fasting is just a way to lose weight or to fight against obesity; however, this is not the only reason to adopt the fasting because it has multiple other health benefits that helps people in multiple way who are following fasting. It includes:

Most importantly, we know that the intermittent fasting has a vital contribution in weight loss. According to the research it is showed up that people who are following the intermittent fasting follow the weight loss more rapidly than those who are not. Thus, it is an effective and quick way to lose weight and control over the calories than any other dieting method.

With intermittent fasting the metabolism function increased and helps with multiple health benefits, such as the reduction of the risk of heart disease, the decrease of the chances of diabetes and the control the blood inflammation Eventually, it is also helpful for obese people.

With good health and fitness, a person can live a long and healthy life. Besides, there is slow process of aging and a reduction of damaging the cell.

Most importantly, according to the health consultants and nutritionist, intermittent fasting is a safe an appropriate way to not only lose weight but also to improve the health. It is a completely new and organized way to have the meals that not only nourished the person health, but also gives a proper diet plans and charts to boost the overall body function.

**Things To Consider Before Starting**

No doubt, intermittent fasting is the best and result oriented way to not only reduce the weight but also improve the overall health condition. Moreover, it is important to know that before fasting, it is not appropriate for everyone, especially for people having some medical issues. Here are some people who cannot do the intermittent fasting, includes:

- Those who are under weight and do not have a healthier maintained body weight.
- If you have a digestive issue or a long history of some eating problem.
- The patients who are suffering from the chronical disease like high blood pressure, heart problem or diabetics. They are not allowed to put themselves on the intermittent fasting. If at any situation they have to do it, then they have to follow a doctor recommendation.
- Women who are pregnant and breastfeeding, are not allowed to follow the intermittent fasting.

That's all because the low calorie or strict diet ratio may be dangerous for such people and could cause different health complications.

Following the intermittent fasting is the challenging task for especially those who want to lose weight by restricting themselves with minimum food. It is a complete change of eating pattern and it sounds difficult to follow in starting. But gradually it becomes easy, it is one of the magical diet-plan that helps to lose weight and improve health without counting the calories. However, according to the health advisors, before starting the intermittent fasting it is essential to consult the doctor, so take the proper advice and follow the respective instructions to get the quick and appropriate outcomes.

# Chapter 8
# Intermittent Fasting And Workout

---

*"It's important to note that our fasting window should be tailored around our workout regimen."*
*Demmy James*

---

Fasting is the diet and meal strictness that a person follows throughout a day without cutting and counting on the calories. People do the fasting for the weight loss, to maintain the overall health and to get the fitness benefits, etc. Intermittent fasting is the new and completely modified form of diet that gets popularity among people, due to multiple of reasons. Some people believe to still follow the workout with the intermittent fasting schedule.

It's not something which can hurt your health, it's just a change in plan to have a meal during the days. There are multiple ways that people adopt to follow the diet, as well as during intermittent fasting it is completely safe to have workouts. The intensity of your workout should be adjustable and as per the health expert advice. According to the research and fitness expert, if you follow the intermittent fasting, then try not to follow the workout with that in parallel. When you are on fasting, the body is already in a position of active metabolism process and workout also boosts the metabolic function. So, combining the both things together may lead to a crash and may not be good for everyone.

On the other hand, people who are following the intermittent fasting and parallel start working out may see significant effects in weight loss. Consequently, it improves the fitness as well as stamina or leads a high level of losing the fats and reduces weight. Workout utilizes energy and muscles take it from the stored body fats and after that the body requires calories to rebuild. So, it is necessary for the intermittent fasting followers that consume more water during or after workout, in order to keep the body hydrated. You can use some kind of electrolyte while doing the exercise as well.

Both fasting and working out together not only improve the metabolism, but is also good for the overall digestive process. The body absorbs more energy and improves the blood circulation that revitalizes the cells and actives the parts of body where the blood or nutrients are not fully supplied, due to inactivity. With intermittent fasting you can have a whole food snacks, instead of having pre-workout meals, because they are good in energy supply and deliver healthy amount of proteins and carbs into the body.

## Fasting And Gain Muscle

Usually, people think and consider that the fasting is the way to lose weight, as well as muscle mass. Thinking in different paradigm, like maintain or gain muscle with intermittent fasting is relatively difficult so, in this process, people put themselves into a strict diet plan and follow limited meal program to get the appropriate results. Limited calorie intake and meal window help to lose weight and to get the lean muscle mass, but is not possible for the muscle gain. For the muscle gain a person needs to consume more calories with the workout that stimulates the tissues growth and increases in overall muscle mass.

### *Weight training in fasting*

Weight trainings are good for the muscle strength and for improving overall stamina. It puts a person metabolism in an active position that leads healthier lifestyle. Intermittent fasting significantly affects the overall weight reduction quickly so, doing the weight training with the fasting, may help to prevent the loss of muscle mass. As per the training professional and health expert, it is highly recommended to do the weight training with the fasting way to lose weight and strengthen the muscles.

***Safety tips during exercise with fasting***

Generally, research supports well to fasting and working out together, but to have great and effective outcomes, it is necessary to follow the way in an appropriate manner that just decreases the weight, not the health, such as doing the exercise with fasting but following the safety tips to combine them in a safe way. Here are some safety tips a person should follow during workouts with intermittent fasting:

In fasting meal timing plays an important role, fitness expert suggests to take a meal close to your workout intensity; this, not only help to fuel up the body with energy, but you can also enjoy the better results with your high intensity workouts.

It is known that during the training it is important to keep the body hydrated, so consume more water during the fasting time and use some electrolytes, which are low calorie source to fuel up muscles and tissues, instead of any energy drink or a workout drink.

Working out with intermittent fasting is good, but parallel a person needs to listen up the body first, as if you follow a high intensity exercise and you feel a kind of exertion, then take a break because it is important.

***Build or maintain muscles***

Intermittent fasting gives the fastest result way of dieting, as long as it is an exceptional way, not like a random method to lose weight. People follow a meal window as per their requirement and fast for a certain time or day in a week; it not only helps to improve the health but is good for losing weight effectively. If you add fasting with working out, the results will be multiplying by two. Remember that the fasting and exercise together just help to give muscle strength and they give quick results, but for gaining the mass it is not an appropriate way because, to gain muscle, usually a person needs to consume more calorie and then burns it through workout. By combining the intermittent fasting with the workout only give a way to maintain the muscle mass and strengthen them.

## Effects On Men & Women Physique

Intermittent fasting is considered as the best way to lose weight and control over the obesity. It is one of the most popular diet-plan that is getting popular, due to its unique and remarkable benefits. If we talk about the effects of the intermittent fasting on men & women, then, according to the studies, it is reported that both have different results and experiences while following the fasting. This is because the hormones and the behaviors change, as well as the results and responses of the body towards the same phenomena.

### *Women struggles more than men*

According to the study, it is reviewed that women struggle more than men in losing the weight and to get the lean muscle mass, because the hormonal changes and chemical reactions are totally changed in both of them. So, intermittent fasting, strict diet and workout plans affect the hormones production and can influence the fertility and reproduction more in women than in men. The women internal system is more sensitive than men's and effects the muscle mass while losing the weight. It can increase the chances of improper ovulation cycle that can disturbed the hormonal balance and cycle.

### *Why women face hormonal deficiencies?*

While following the intermittent fasting, women face the hormonal deficiency that may cause multiple of health complications like indigestion problem, disturbed menstruation cycle and effect, due to the loss of muscle mass with the weight and fats. Other than a man, a woman faces more problems because she's not able to take the proteins and, due to strict diet and meal plans, hormonal changes occur and affect them more rapidly.

There are multiple of reasons a woman can face problems with fasting, like:

- Low level of nutrients and consumption of the food may cause the nutrients deficiency.
- If a woman follows tight and high intensity workouts with the fasting, they are followed the too much stress and exertion.
- It can be due to limited time for the recovery and rest between the workouts and fasting breakouts.

- Low level of the intake can affect the immune system and raise the chances of illness like flu, fever, infection and others.

### *How stress influence health and hormonal level?*

When a person on the low carbs and calorie diet, has to definitely face multiple of hormonal and behavioral changes. Sometimes people are too aggressive towards the following of the intermittent fasting meal window with the exercise, so the result is stress and undue pressure to lose weight quickly that significantly affect their ability to fight against the upcoming challenges. High level of stress hormones production disturbs the balance of hormonal level and disturbs overall function abruptly.

The most important thing in this situation that has to be considered is consulting the health consultant and making a meal plan accordingly. Be consistent in following the plan, do not stress out to get quick results, listen to your body and act accordingly. Eat the healthy and nutritional food with the low or high intensity workout and follow the guideline of the instructor and health consultant to avoid the issue.

## Best Exercise During Intermittent Fasting

Workout is the best way to keep yourself active, as well as it has a vital effect on the person's overall health. With regular exercise you can not only enjoy a fresh and lively lifestyle, but also it boosts the metabolism function. By an improved blood circulation many health complications can be deal in a better way. If a person follows a diet plan to lose weight, then combining the workout could significantly impact the overall results; even the researchers recommend that intermittent fasting can be more useful and beneficial if it is followed by a proper schedule exercise. It can be high or low intensity trainings as per the person's capability and requirements.

The choice of the trainings depends on the method of intermittent fasting that a person chooses to lose weight. In general, it's just a followed meal plans a person adopts for a day to lose the excessive weight, so it does not only improve the health but it also elicits other complications that can influence a person's life, due to obesity.

### *Workout timings with fasting*

For the right and fruitful results, it is necessary to follow the right way to involve the workout plans. For example, some people follow the two times working out routine with the intermittent fasting and others have one; this depends on the method you choose for fasting and the intensity you want to have to get the results, so the morning time is considered an appropriate time to work out with fasting.

### *Build your own workout routine*

You can follow or build your own workout routine as well; aforementioned, it depends on what you are expecting from your body to be followed. Some people want to lean muscle mass and reduce the size, others are looking to reduce the fats or weight by gaining the muscle mass. You can build or design your own workout routine that entirely depends on the priority you are looking for. Firstly, for the muscle mass adopt the weight training with the cardio sessions and consume more proteins that give strength to the muscle. Secondly, for strength deadlifts, push-ups, dips, pull ups and squats are considered effective workouts for women and men as well.

### *Weight trainings with fasting*

Weight training with intermittent fasting is an effective option because it will not only help to lose weight, but it will also improve the stamina, strength for the muscle growth. Sometimes people may lose the muscle weight while following the intermittent fasting plans, so the weight training will keep the muscle in shape and do not let you lose the mass.

### *Cardio session with fasting*

Cardio sessions are not only effective for weight lose but also help to improve the blood circulation throughout the body. These sessions help to keep a person active and considered more effective to have a good stamina and strength; with fasting it will help to improve the overall metabolic process and reduce inflammation in blood and body.

### *Cardiovascular exercises*

Cardiovascular trainings are effective and can be done anywhere like at gym or at home; you do not need a special gym equipment. These trainings are effective and 25 times more effective then pulling and pushing weights. Leg raises, crunches, squats, push-ups, pull-ups etc. are effective and influential trainings that can be done with fasting to get the healthier outcomes.

# Chapter 9
## Tips For Successful Transformation



Losing weight and being back in the ideal physique is a challenging job for people who are dealing with the obesity issue. But in reality, there is nothing that cannot be possible in real life. As a matter of fact, there are multiple of diet plans and health tips that are really helpful and impressive to give the outcomes with no side effects. Intermittent fasting is considered one of them, it is not like any other traditional way to diet and lose fats, as it provides a meal window between the fasting: eating and fasting are divided in between the whole day. This method boosts metabolism and helps to transform the body.

If you are one of those who is tired of the weight and fats or wants to lose them effectively to be back in a good shape, then intermittent fasting is the appropriate and impressive way to be active and fit without any health side effects. It is getting popular because it provides ease and comfort in life with the simple window of fasting and eating in a day. According to the health professionals, it is important to follow the procedure for at least one or two months continuously, without any break.

People who followed the fasting methods talked about this proudly and discussed their body transformation. To achieve the ideal and fit body with lean muscle mass, it is necessary to follow some impressive tips and procedure that will not only help to reduce the weight, as well strengthen the overall muscle mass with the strong and impressive way.

## Motivational Success Stories

Losing weight and being back in the fit and slim physique is quite difficult and tough. There are multiple of people around us who tried multiple ways to do that but failed. Losing weight is not something a magic can happen to anyone in a day or weeks, it leads a continues change or lifestyle change that brings hope and transformation. Intermittent fasting is getting popular among people around the world just because of its remarkable benefits and long-term benefits in a person's life.

If we just look around, we can easily find multiple success stories, who just tried and lost weight with following the intermittent fasting meal windows. Here we have some for you to just give a motivation and inspiration to follow:

1. James Kevin

By profession James is a doctor, he guides others about the health, fitness and leading good lifestyle, but due to his unwanted eating habits and food choice made him fat. He even did not think to get back into to shape, then an incident happened in his life that changed everything completely. His sister died with a serious chronical disease, right at that movement he realized that he had an option. Indeed, with the intermittent fasting he put himself in the stick schedule of eating vegetables and low carbs food product and followed a proper workout session parallel to the fasting; the results were amazing in just 18 months: he lost around 125 pounds.

"I am amazed with the results, there are diets that give results but intermittent fasting is medically an amazing one. That's why I choose this and see the difference." James Kevin

2. Jane Wright

Being a mother is no doubt a blessing, but a person has to go along with the whole process of fighting for the weight loss.

Jane got a lot of weight after having a baby and tried multiple ways to reduce but failed. The motivation she had to be the perfect and fit mother by physique, as well as her daughter can be proud of her. With the weight of 337 pounds she just started the intermitted fasting 21-day meal plan. Parallel to this, she added the 30 minutes cardio training session into her routine that went for the high intensity workouts. She fasted for almost 16 hours a day and only eat 8 hours; with all her effects and dedication, she just lost the 105 pounds in 12 months. She shared her excitement: "I am happy and motivated and found quality time with my daughter like never before. With this, all I have patience and consistency, which are the keys to achieve any of your goals."

3. Hunter Hobbs

He is a man with weight of almost 200 pounds with the height of 5 feet 10 inches. He found himself overweight and decided to choose the meal plan of intermittent fasting, with the continuous effort of three months, the consistent fasting, eating meal windows and workouts he almost lost the 42 pounds. He takes picture of himself every day and tracks his all way of transformation together. He just lost the almost 42 pounds in three months with the intermittent fasting meal plans.

He was excited and he shared his review, "I am surprised and amazed with the results of this intermittent fasting. I just started following this by getting the inspiration from the multiple people who shared their success stories. This gave me encouragement to make myself as an inspiration for someone."

## 4. Brittany May

Brittany May was a woman with the weight of 514 pounds and she was getting hard for her to handle it all together. She heard about the intermittent fasting meal plans and she chose the one for herself. With the continuous effort of following the diet plan and exercise, she reduced almost 336 pounds in the period of two years. It is an incredible achievement as May said, "I actually want to lose the stubborn body weight and change my lifestyle to enjoy the pleasure of lifestyle and relationship, now finally I got what I want to get." Losing weight not only transformed her life, but also gave her a new direction to drive it on her own way.

## 5. Ria Reed

Intermittent fasting proven the best and most comfortable way to lose weight and get lean muscle mass. Ria lost almost 32 pounds with the transformed body mass; thanks to the intermitted fasting, with the high intensity cardio session and weight trainings, she did not only achieve her target, but she also felt confident about sharing her transformation path.

She shares that the "the family holidays become memorable and more than expectations than I never had in dreams before."

6. Kelly and Mike

Losing weight together is a couple goals that is proved by Kelly and Mike. Both give motivation to each other's and started the intermittent fasting together. At the starting time Kelly was with the weight of 219 pounds and Mike have weight 259 pounds. After eating or fasting with 21 days' meal plan and exercise, both lost some remarkable pounds like Kelly lost 57 pounds and Mike lost 58 pounds. That was an incredible change for both of them, so that they shared their motivational and transformation story together.

## Tips For Transformation

While following the fasting, people achieve their body transformation target with the impressive way within time. According to the experiences of different people, multiple things are really important and they boost the process to achieve the targets really quickly. Transformation needs the working and strict to the plan with the proper discipline and dedication. If you follow fasting, it does not mean you do not need planning. Making strategy and the implementation of a right plan to achieve right outcomes is an important and necessary option.

Here we have some impressive tips for those who are new and want to follow the transformation procedure to get an impressive body.

### Remove junk food

Most important thing that a person has to consider for the body transformation, is that she / he has to remove all the junk food from the house, because fasting, initially, makes it is difficult to fight from the hunger, and in case of hunger attack there are probabilities to consume the junk, if they are in approach. So, replace the junk food with the healthy snacks and whole food that are full of protein and low in carbs, this it helps to make your stomach feel full for a longer time and makes things easier at the time of the fasting.

### Interact socially

If you are facing problem with fighting obesity in its best way, then it is important to fight and interact with the social circle, for example: ask friends, family and other close ones to how and what to follow for the transformation, because around us it is easy to find out the impressive stories of people who have done lots of efforts on themselves, and their experiences could support other people.

### Start reading about food and health

Reading will definitely give impressive ideas and awareness about the things in totally different way. Firstly, for the successful transformation a person needs to start reading about the other's successful stories to get the motivation. Secondly, a person needs to find out more about the food and things that helps to boost metabolism and what to avoid if someone wants to achieve a desired fit and slim physique.

### Have picture before starting

The necessary thing before starting the fasting or any other method of diet is to take a picture and save it as a record; this will give a motivation to go long on the way of fasting or dieting, and helps to track the performance too.

### Be consistent with plan

Consistency is more than necessary in the way that a person chooses to go along with, as it is not about that you just start for some time and then switch to another plan. So, for the intermittent fasting, it is important to at least try the method for one or two months consecutively.

### Bring changes into workout routine

Workout really helps in the whole transformation process, it gives muscles strength and put the body in the process of continuous fat reduction. If a person is following a low and simple intensity workout, then it is necessary to move towards the high intensity workout schedule and modify the trainings. Consequently, you can add the weight trainings and high intensity cardio trainings in the whole routine to get the better outcomes.

### Plan and prepare meal

Consume more green vegetables and protein in your daily intake with the exercise and other activities; try to prepare the whole food with low fats and low carbs options. Watching out on the fat intake is another important thing for the transformation, use the nuts as a source of good fats, but check the calories you are consuming in your eating time.

### Improve the self-control

During the whole process of fasting or dieting the difficult things is to keep the check on the hand and the choice of having the meals all around, as long as a person may face the episodes of the hunger and craving. Thus, improve your self-control over the junk by choosing the healthy and low carbs food option and switch to whole food instead of high carbs, and so on. Furthermore, clean your snacks choices or meal at the time of eating so you can survive best at the time of fasting.

### Keep yourself hydrated

Hydration is the most important consideration; during workouts and meal plans consume more water and low calories drinks options. Water helps to keep up the metabolism that actively boosts the process of fat reduction and helps in transformation. So, tea, coffee, electrolytes and other non-sugary drinks can be consumed in the fasting or with the eating schedule as well.

### Manage stress

Stress can be a hurdle in the whole process of transformation. Thus, it is important to reduce the stress and keep the control on it, because it could affect the process of weight loss and fats reduction. Lastly, to lower the stress, try to have good amount of sleep and rest after workouts and between the exercises.

### Set goals and share

Without goals, setting the process cannot be measured so fast. To get the impressive transformation try to make a defined goal, such as short term goals and share them with your social circle; this will help to keep up the motivational level and a courage to achieve them in the short time period.

Whatever the procedure you are following for the transformation like intermittent fasting or any other diet plan, the important thing is to keep following with a consistent time period. Consistency is the key to achieve any of the goal, whether it is related to the health and fitness target. Intermittent fasting is getting popular because of its impressive and outstanding results that are not only to reduce the weight, but also to give multiple other health benefits.

# Chapter 10
# **Women And Intermittent Fasting**

Intermittent fasting is the most popular method if you want to get the lean muscle mass and to reduce the weight. A person who is following this way to diet have a more energetic and motivated journey to lose weight. Intermittent fasting will defiantly give multiple health benefits, no matter you are a man or a woman. The important consideration is just that every person has different biological structure, so things will work differently for everyone. Some can get the results quickly and others have to stay and consistent for a little longer to get the results. But generally, it is the safe and best way to lose weight. However, according to the multiple research, the intermittent fasting is highly recommendable for men but not for women.

Intermittent fasting is a bit technical method that works by engaging the body in the process of absorbing and digestion of food into the body and keeps the body fuel up for the whole time of fasting. Besides, it accelerates the process of fats burning in the state of fasting; in simple words, fasting is the period that usually there are around 12, 16 or 18 hours of fasting, in which you should not have food or just consume water or low- calorie drinks like green tea, coffee or tea without sugar and milk. Usually people have the meal window of around 8 hours or 6 hours a day and the rest of the time spend on fasting.

## What's good with intermittent fasting?

Intermittent fasting is an effective result and is oriented to diet and to lose weight, by giving remarkable good outcomes, which are:

- Loss weight and it helps to maintain the healthy one
- With this it is easy to get the lean muscle mass and muscle strength as well
- A person can feel energetic and can control over the junk food
- It can increase the insulin sensitivity and reduce the inflammation
- It also helps to enhance the overall cognitive function

## Intermittent fasting sounds tricky for women

In general, intermittent fasting is an impressive and technical thing to lose weight but for women it is a way different thing. It happens because the woman system is different from man's and production or responses of the hormones to a certain scenario is totally changed. The intense fasting with the workout not only leans the muscle mass, but it also makes changes in hormones. Especially, it affects directly on the fertility hormones and ovulation process. Due to hormonal disturbance a woman can experience multiple health issues like:

- Irregular menstruation cycle
- Metabolic stress and anxiety
- Fertility issues
- Ovulation disturbance
- Difficult to take enough or good sleep
- Ovaries can be shrinking and make difficult to conceive

If a woman wants to follow the intermittent fasting then most importantly, make sure to follow the relax and different fasting and eating approach. It can be convenient if the method must be chosen after consulting the health consultant, so the hormones function will not be disturbed.

## During Mensuration

For a woman it is technical and crucial to follow a diet plan to lose the weight, as compared to men. Because both have different hormones and behaviors of the hormones that respond differently in different situations. In general studies it is not sure that the intermittent fasting can cause problems with the menstruation cycle, but it can in some cases. In fasting usually people lower the calories intake that turns it an effective way to overcome the metabolic problem and reduce the weight; nonetheless, causing issue with the periods does not just happen because of the intermittent fasting.

According to some studies, it is discussed that the intermittent fasting can influence the periods in a woman, if the calorie intake reduces up to a drastic low level, because fasting puts the body in the high metabolic process and, due to lower calorie diet and narrow eating window, it effects the hormones production. Finally, imbalance hormones directly influence the fertility and menstruation.

The important thing that need to be considered while following intermittent fasting is add nutrients in your eating window like nuts, fruits, green leafy vegetables and a lot of healthy snacks, as long as they will keep the body function streamline to act properly, and they also help to control over the exertion and stressful condition that can influence the hormonal balance badly.

## For Pregnancy & Breastfeeding

In women, hormones are interconnected and influence by the intense internal deficiencies that can cause low calorie intake or low nutritional food supply to the cells and body parts; with intermittent fasting, metabolism function goes high and utilizes the internal stored energy to keep the energy level up. However, if due to intense fasting and exertion hormones got disturbed, they lead to the disturbance in the digestion, metabolism, blood pressure or blood sugar level as well. So, the adverse situation can be the cause of infertility, improper periods session or other fertility issues.

Health consultant does not suggest the intermittent fasting to those women who is trying to conceive or pregnant ones. As well as breastfeeding mothers, they should follow the intermittent fasting because it can affect the nutrients and energy components that are essential for a child in the early ages.

Losing weight is good, but a person needs to listen up the body first, such as for pregnant and breastfeeding women, it is not suitable to mess up with the hormonal production just to lose the weight.


## During Menopause

Menopause is the process that a woman has to face and goes through in the early age like around 40 or 50. During the process multiple health and hormonal changes take place inside the body that effect the body structure and hormonal changes equally.

## *What Is menopause?*

It is a period that a woman does not have periods for the entire year or more than that, it happens when the ovaries stop producing the eggs. Usually, an average ratio of menopause occurs at the age of 45 or 51 years; it is considered as a hard time and multiple health complications can affect a woman, for instance: a woman is not able to conceive when the procedure begins and gradually stops the periods that leads high level of hormonal and behavioral changes.

## *How menopause effect a woman life?*

During the process of menopause, the body produces limited amount of progesterone or testosterone hormones. High level of hormonal changes can have multiple effects on a person's life, such as:

- Gaining weight and fats quickly
- Facing the stress and high level of anxiety
- Due to low testosterone sex driving can be affected, as well as facing vaginal dryness
- Sometime facing hair loss, mood swings and dry skin issues
- Insomnia and restless sleeping

## *Menopause and weight*

Menopause directly affects the weight, usually it is noticed that woman gains weight quickly, due to the certain body and hormonal changes in the body. Furthermore, there are multiple other factors that can influence the overall health, such as the increase in weight that can develop the risk of obesity and high blood pressure. Parallel, it may have disturbed the blood glucose level in the body that can increase the risk of diabetes.

Due to certain complications and problems, doctors highly recommend to control over the weight gain and try to adopt the ways to reduce it with the optimal level, by means of proper schedule diet and workout sessions that can only give opportunity to control the weight and other associated issues. A hormonal test is recommended as well.

### *Intermitted fasting in menopause*

Intermittent fasting is the tested and highly recommended way to lose the weight and it restores the energy and stamina. It is followed by extended the time between the meals and fasting, as the glucose is the primary source of the energy that your body needs to function properly. While with fasting, the body is not able to get the glucose from the food and it starts getting it from the stored body fats; in the end, it gradually starts burning the fats and utilizes that energy to spend the hours of fasting.

Health consultants consider that a woman during the menopause can adopt the intermittent fasting technique to lose weight and to fuel up the body energy, for the reason that it does not only keep you out of stress, but it also manages the insulin level, reduces inflammation and is good for the overall cognitive function. The ideal hours of fasting for a day is 16 hours or 12 hours and between the meal window of 6 hours or 8 hours; During the eating time it is important to consume excessive water, as well as during the fasting time.

## The Best Methods Of Intermittent Fasting For Women

Intermittent fasting is considered a technical concept that needs a lot of effort to measure the exact fasting and eating ratio, so the health complications can be avoided. Experts said that the intensity of fasting for women cannot be the same as for men, this is because each of them has different hormonal functions that leads in a body differently. As well as the biological structure of both of them is totally different from each other, so, it is important to avoid the fasting, if you may face the serious health complication and, due to any reason, face some significant side effects.

### *Tips to adopt for fasting*

By considering the health and hormonal changes a woman has to follow the tips that are designed and prescribed by the experts. It includes:

- Try not to follow the intense fasting schedule like do not fast for more than 24 hours at once.

- The best time zone and schedule to fast is 12 hours or probably 16 hours

- Do not fast for consecutive days in the first two or three weeks of fasting, always try to indulge with the alternative days for fasting.

- Keep your self-hydrated during the whole fasting time and follow the good nutritional food to break-fast.

- Do not go for the intense training or the weight trainings, especially in the days of fasting, the best training sessions are like yoga, light cardio, walking or running which are the appropriate options.

- Break your fast if you feel dizziness or any unpleasant feeling during the fasting.

- Keep yourself fuel up in eating hours with the good fats like nuts, low carb diet and proteins, because they are good in weight loss, as well as maintain the hormonal balance.

There are multiple of fasting methods that are common and popular among the people, but due to the biological structure differences, every method is not appropriate for women. However, that doesn't mean a woman cannot fast to lose weight, though there are some effective and useful ways that are feasible and appropriate for them. Plus, they do not harm the hormonal balances and they never cause the fertility issues.

Here are some methods for the safe intermittent fasting for women:

### 16:8 method

This is one of the most popular and common method of intermittent fasting. The method is also known as the lean-gains method. This way not only helps to reduce the weight but it is also effective to get the lean muscle mass. This method is considered completely safe for the women. Finally, in this intermittent fasting, an individual follows the 16 hours of having fast and 6 hours for eating throughout a day.

### 24-hour protocol

It is another effective and safe intermitted fasting method for women that usually follows just twice in a week: it is also known as eat-stop-eat fasting type. Usually in this fasting type a person does not have any eating window and has to follow the 24 hours of fast. According to the health consultant for woman, it is necessary to just follow this method twice a week, but more than that may be not good for the health.

### 5:2 diet plan

5:2 diet plan is the fast diet in which a person has to divide the meal into two equal parts with just 500 calorie consumption in a day. This diet is just followed two days in a week and rest of the day you can take normal food. This fast diet is considered the safe one for both men and women. You can have two days with the meal of 500 calories for each day and the rest of five days a week follow the normal diet.

# Chapter 11: Recipes

## *Best Breakfast Recipes*

## Raspberry Power Pancake

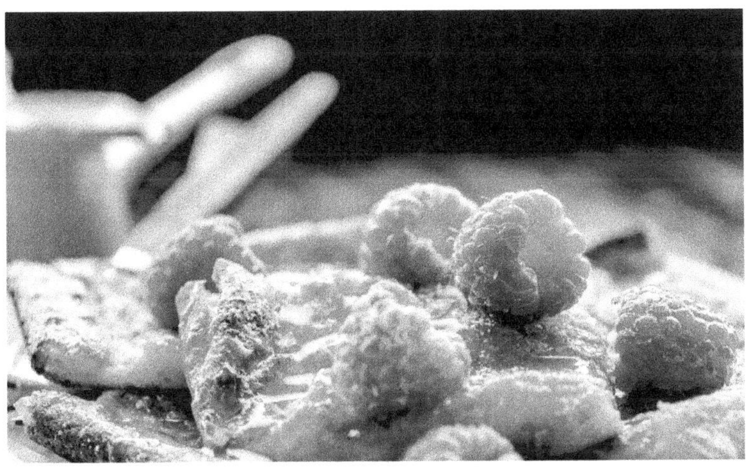

***Preparation time****: 05 minutes | **Cooking time***: *15 minutes | **Servings***: *4*

**Ingredients:**

- 1 egg
- 1 and 1/3 cups flour
- ¼ teaspoon vanilla extract
- 2 tablespoons
- melted butter
- 1 ½ cups milk
- ½ teaspoon salt

- 3 teaspoons baking powder
- 2 tablespoons vegetable oil
- 1 tablespoon ground sugar
- 1 cup raspberries

**Directions:** Mix egg, milk, vanilla extract, and butter in a bowl. Mix flour, salt and baking powder in another bowl. Now add these mixed dry ingredients into the egg batter. Mix it well and leave it for 5 minutes. Preheat the pan on medium flame. Grease the pan with vegetable oil. Pour the 1/4$^{th}$ batter into the pan and add raspberries at the top. Cook it for few minutes until bubbles start to appear. Now flip it and cook the other side for 2 minutes. Sprinkle the grounded sugar on the pancakes.

**Nutrition:** Protein 8g, Calories 329, Fat 14g, Carbohydrate 46g.

# Chocolate Chip Whey Waffles

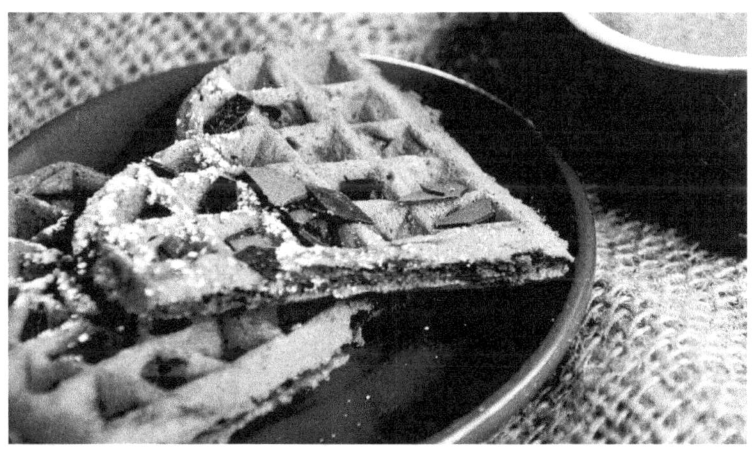

***Preparation time***: *10 minutes* | ***Cooking time***: *10 minutes* | ***Servings***: *2*

## Ingredients:

- 2 eggs
- 1 tablespoon baking powder
- 2 tablespoons coconut flour
- 2 scoop chocolate whey protein
- ½ tablespoon vanilla extract
- 1 tablespoon coconut sugar
- 1 tablespoon chocolate chips

## Directions:

Preheat the greased waffle iron. In a bowl mix flour, protein powder, sugar, and baking powder. Now add rest of the ingredients in the dry mixture and mix them until all the ingredients combined properly. Now put the batter in the preheated waffle iron and cook for approximately 4 minutes. Serve it immediately by adding some chocolate chips on its top.

**Nutrition:** Protein 28g, fat 9g, Carbohydrate 25g, Calories 292, Sugar 14g, Cholesterol 228mg.

# Cinnamon Sugar Donuts

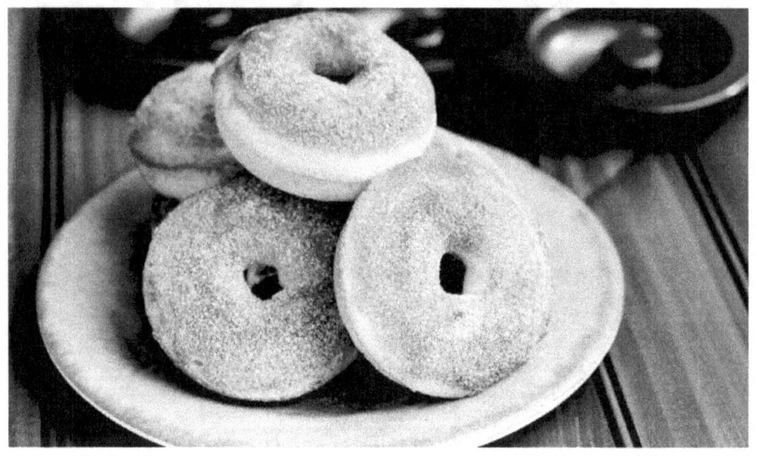

*Preparation time: 10 minutes | **Cooking time**: 10 minutes | **Servings**: 2*

## Ingredients:

- ½ cup sugar
- 1 ½ cups flour
- ½ teaspoon salt
- ½ cup milk
- ½ teaspoons cinnamon
- ½ teaspoon nutmeg

- 1 egg
- 1 tablespoon melted butter
- 2 teaspoons baking powder

**Directions:**

Put the mix the salt, flour, nutmeg, baking powder, and cinnamon in a bowl. Take another bowl and mix all the remaining ingredients. Now combine the wet ingredients in the dry ingredients and whisk them well. Take a pan with oil and put the batter in the form of donuts in the oil. Fry these donuts on the medium flame. And serve it immediately.

**Nutrition:** Protein 3.6g, Fat 8.1g, Carbohydrate 34.3g, Calories 222, Sugar 18.6g, Cholesterol 47mg.

# Poached Eggs & Avocado

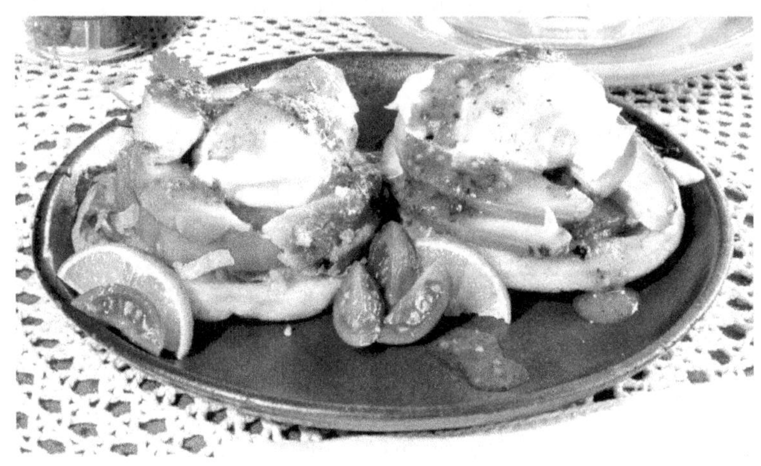

*Preparation time*: 10 minutes I *Cooking time*: 10 minutes I *Servings*: 2

## Ingredients:

- 2 slices of bread
- 2 eggs
- A pinch of salt and black pepper
- 2 tablespoons sheared cheese
- 1/3 smashed avocado
- ½ cup fresh herbs
- ½ cup cubed cut tomatoes

## Directions:

Take a pot to boil the water. Boil the water and turn off the heat. Now carefully crack the eggs in the boiled water. Cover the pot for around 4 to 5 minutes. Toast the bread slices and set the avocado on it. Take out the eggs carefully with the help of a spatula and place it on the toast. Sprinkle salt, pepper, cheese, tomato, and fresh herbs on the egg. And it is ready to serve.

**Nutrition:** Protein 23.3g, Fats 20.4g, Calories 393, Sugar 5.7g, Cholesterol 34.6mg.

# Chocolate Chia Plain Pudding

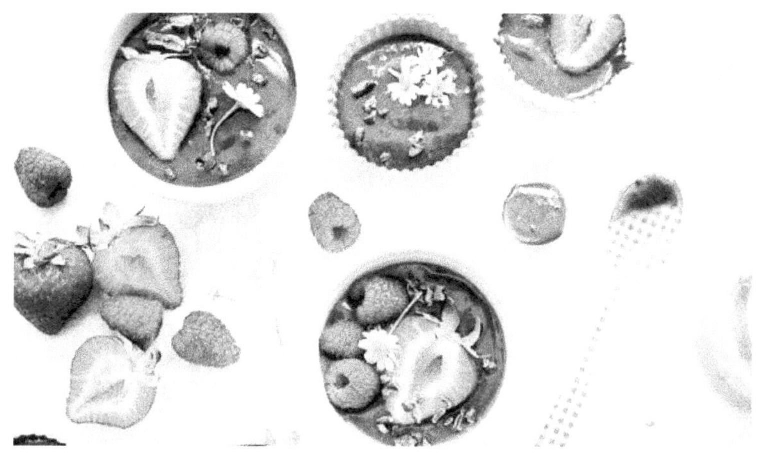

*Preparation time: 05 minutes I **Chilling time**: 4 hours I **Servings**: 2*

**Ingredients:**
- 1/3 cup chia seeds
- 1 cup coconut or almond milk
- ¼ cup cocoa powder
- ½ teaspoon vanilla extract
- 2 tablespoons maple syrup

- ½ cup Seasonal Berries (optional)

**Directions:**

Take a bowl and add all the ingredients in it. Mix all the ingredients until they merged in a proper way. Check the sweet and if required add more syrup in it to make it according to your taste. Now place it in the refrigerator for at least 4 hours for chilling. Serve it by adding berries on its top.

**Nutrition:** Protein 6g, Fats 20.4g, Calories 164, Sugar 1g, Carbohydrates 14g.

# Gluten-Free Pumpkin Pancake

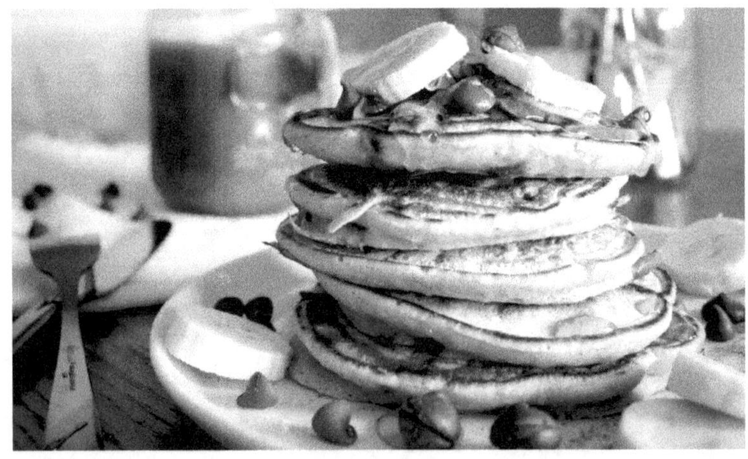

*Preparation time*: 15 minutes | *Cooking time*: 10 minutes | *Servings*: 15

## Ingredients:

- 2 eggs
- 1½ cups low-fat milk
- 2 tablespoons melted butter
- ½ cup pumpkin pure
- 2 teaspoons pumpkin pie spice
- 1 teaspoon vanilla extract
- 1½ cups gluten free pancake mix

## Directions:

Mix eggs, milk, pumpkin puree, and butter in a bowl. Add pancake mix in it gradually and mix it well, salt and baking powder in another bowl. Now add the remaining ingredients and mix well. Put a greased skillet over medium heat and pour better in it. Cook it until its color turned into gold. Cook on both sides and serve it immediately.

**Nutrition:** Protein 3g, Calories 113, Fat 3g, Carbohydrate 19g, Sugar 5g.

# Roasted Sweet Potato & Poblano Tacos

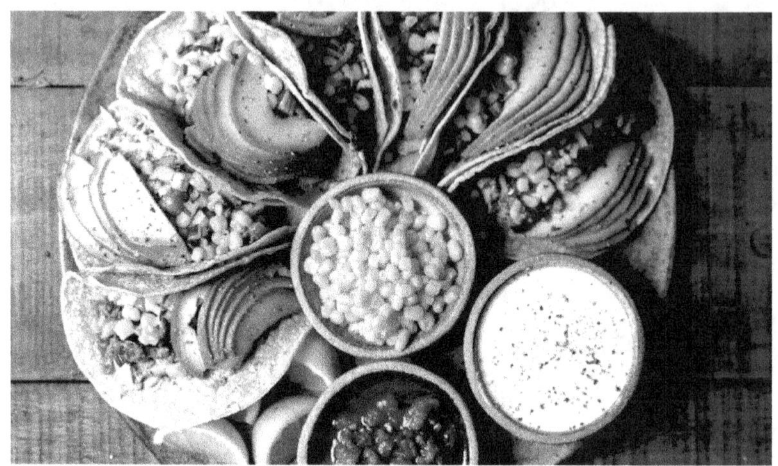

*Preparation time*: 15 minutes | *Cooking time*: 45 minutes | *Servings*: 2

## Ingredients:

- 3 eggs
- 1 cubes sweet potato
- 1 thin sliced pepper bells
- 1 cup corns
- 4 tortillas
- ½ diced avocado
- ½ teaspoon crushed salt and black pepper
- roasted Tomatillo salsa

## Directions:

Preheat the oven at 450F and prepare the baking dish with paper. Roast the salsa and vegetables for 15 minutes into the preheated oven. Now reduce the oven temperature to 425F. Take 2 baking dishes add potatoes in one. And other vegetables in the second. Drizzle oil, salt, and pepper on it and baked potatoes for 25 minutes and vegetables for 15 minutes. Cook eggs and scrambled them. In the serving dish add everything and serve with salsa.

**Nutrition:** Protein 8g, Fat 12g, Carbohydrate 55g, Calories 350, Sugar 10g

# Sugar-Free Oatmeal Cookies

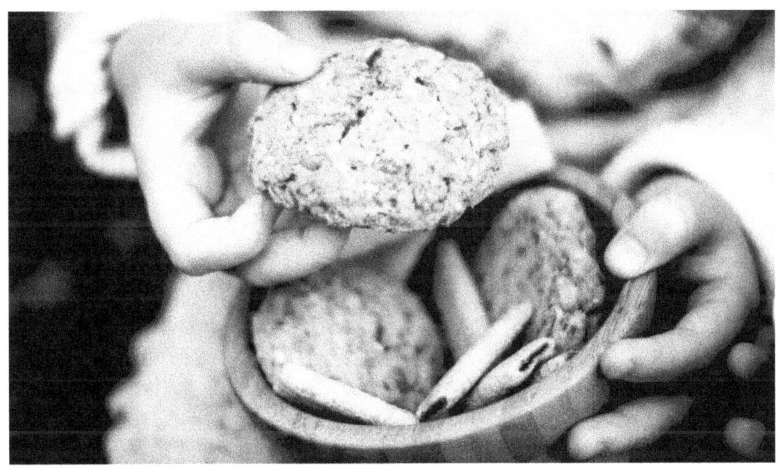

*Preparation time: 10 minutes I **Cooking time**: 10 minutes I **Servings**: 15*

**Ingredients:**
- ½ cup butter

- 2 eggs
- 1 ¼ rolled oats
- 1 teaspoon almond flour
- 1 teaspoon cinnamon
- 1 sugar-free baking powder
- ¼ teaspoon salt
- 1 teaspoon vanilla extract
- ¾ cup of gluten sugar

**Directions:**

Preheat the oven at 350F and prepare a baking tray with a liner. Take a bowl and combine the eggs, butter and gluten sugar and mix well. Now mix the remaining ingredients in it and mix well. Add some water if required to thin the batter so that all the ingredients merged well. Now scoop the batter in the tray and baked it for 10 minutes. It is ready to serve.

**Nutrition:** Protein 3g, Fat 8g, Calories 103g, Carbohydrates 5g, Sugar 0.4g

# Egg Muffin With Broccoli

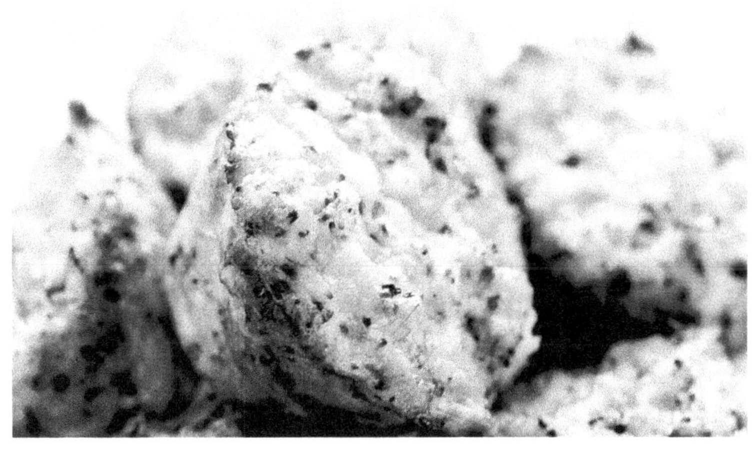

*Preparation time*: *05 minutes* | ***Cooking time***: *15 minutes* | ***Servings***: *12*

## Ingredients:

- 1 teaspoon salt
- 10 eggs
- ½ teaspoon black pepper
- ½ teaspoon garlic powder
- ½ teaspoon thyme
- 2/3 cup grated cheese
- 1½ cups steamed and chopped broccoli

## Directions:

Prepare 12 muffin cups with liner and preheat the oven at 400F temperature. Take a bowl and beat the eggs thoroughly. Now add the remaining ingredients in it by adding cheese and broccoli in the last. Mix all the ingredients until they merged well. Pour the batter in the prepared muffin cups evenly. Bake it for 12 to 15 minutes and serve it immediately.

**Nutrition:** Protein 6g, Fats 5g, Calories 82, Cholesterol 142mg.

# Banana Blueberry Muffins

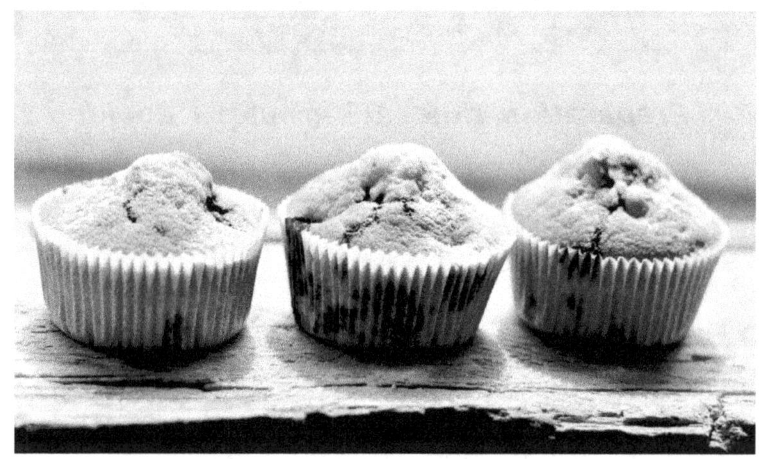

***Preparation time****: 10 minutes | **Cooking time***: 20 minutes | ***Servings****: 12*

## Ingredients:

- 1 egg
- 1/2 cup mashed banana
- ¼ cup vegetable oil
- 2/3 cup milk
- 2/3 cup gluten sugar
- 2½ cup teaspoons baking powder

- 2 cups flour
- 1 cup well drained blueberries

**Directions:** Take a bowl and add all the ingredients except blueberries. Stir it well until all the ingredients merged. In the end, add blueberries in it and fold it in the mixture. Prepare the 12 muffin cups with liner. Pour the batter equally in the cups. Put the cups in the 400F temperature preheated oven for 18 to 20 minutes. Your muffins are ready.

**Nutrition:** Protein 4.5g, Fats 10g, Calories 332, Sugar 31g, Carbohydrates 58g.

## Grilled Cheeseburger

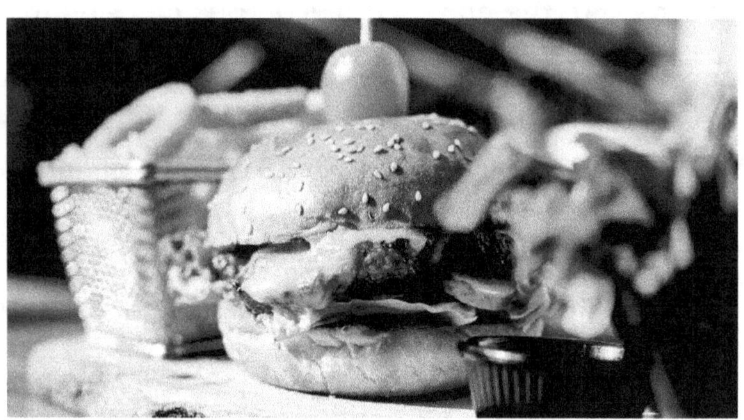

*Preparation time: 15 minutes | Cooking time: 15 minutes | Servings: 4*

**Ingredients:**

- 2 chopped tomatoes
- 1 tablespoon olive oil
- 1 cup taco seasoning
- 3 tablespoons unsalted butter
- 1 ½ cup grated cheese
- 8 slices wheat bread
- ½ teaspoon salt and black pepper
- 1 pound ground beef

**Directions:** Put a skillet with oil over the medium flame. Cook the beef by adding salt and pepper in it for 5 minutes until it cooked well. Add cheese, tomato, and seasoning in it and cook it for about 1 minute until cheese melted. Take the bread and apply butter on it and grill it. Now spread the beef better on the 4 slices evenly and add cheese on it. Cover it with the second slice and it is ready to serve.

**Nutrition:** Protein 42.8g, Fats 43.2g, Calories 701.4, Sugar 6.6g, Carbohydrates 35.7g, Cholesterol 140.8mg.

# Asian Chicken Salad

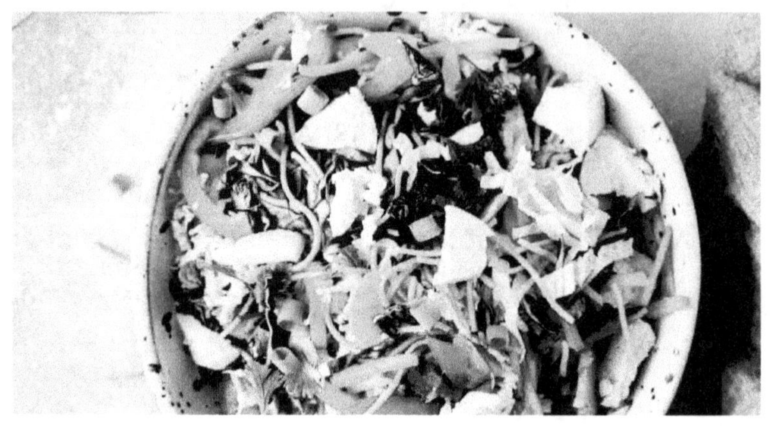

*Preparation time*: 20 minutes | *Cooking time*: 10 minutes | *Servings*: 6

## Ingredients:

- 1 thinly sliced red bell pepper
- 1 peeled and sliced carrot
- 2 thinly sliced chicken breasts
- 1 shredded lettuce
- 1 shredded cabbage
- ½ teaspoon salt and black pepper
- 2 tablespoons chopped basil leaves
- ½ cup toasted almonds
- 2 tablespoons soy sauce
- 2 tablespoons grated sugar
- ¼ cup vegetable oil
- 1 tablespoon vinegar

**Directions:** Grill the thinly sliced chicken. Take a bowl and add bell pepper, carrot, grilled chicken, lettuce, cabbage, basil, almonds, salt, and pepper. Mix all the ingredients well. Now for dressing mix sauce, sugar, vinegar, and vegetable in a bowl. Pour it over the salad and present it.

**Nutrition:** Protein 15.1g, Fats 8.1g, Calories 210, Sugar 6g, Carbohydrates 20g, Cholesterol 21mg

## Keto Chicken Lettuce Wraps

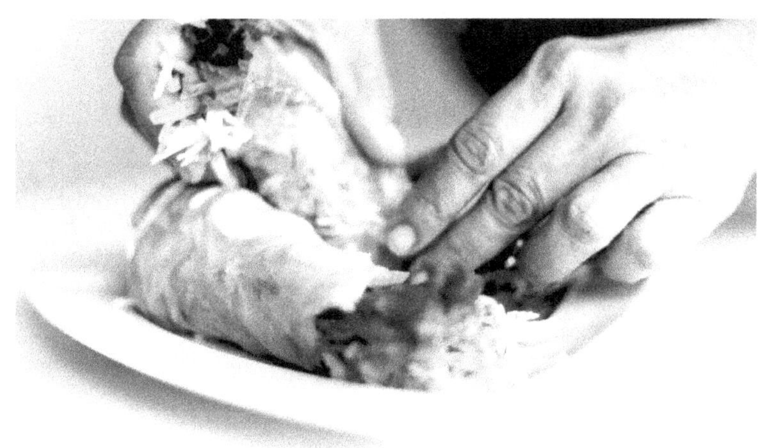

*Preparation time: 10 minutes | Cooking time: 15 minutes | Servings: 12*

**Ingredients:**
- 2 shredded chicken breasts

- 1 cup diced tomatoes
- ½ teaspoon salt
- ½ teaspoon black pepper
- 1 sliced green onion
- 1 diced avocado
- ½ cup grated cheese
- 2 teaspoons lemon juice
- 12 leaves of lettuce

**Directions:**

In a pan boil the shredded chicken for around 15 minutes. Take a bowl and add all the ingredients leaving lettuce leaves. Add the boiled and shredded chicken in it as well and mix all the ingredients thoroughly. Take lettuce leaves and put a small amount of batter on all the leaves and wrap them. Serve it cold.

**Nutrition:** Protein 9g, Fats 5g, Calories 93, Carbohydrates 2g, Cholesterol 29mg, Fiber 1g.

# Egg And Vegetable Bagel Sandwich

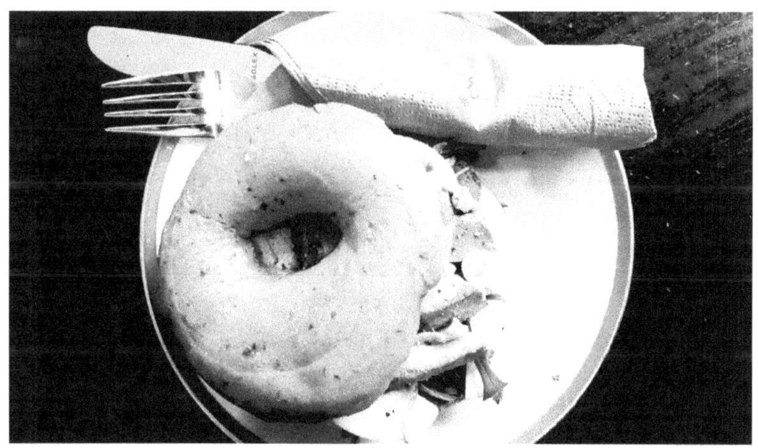

**Preparation time**: 05 minutes | **Cooking time**: 05-07 minutes | **Servings**: 1

## Ingredients:

- 1 thin bagel
- 1 tablespoon olive oil
- 2 sliced mushrooms
- ½ sliced avocado
- ½ cup crushed spinach leaves
- 2 eggs whites
- ½ cup cubed tomatoes
- ½ cup diced red pepper
- A pinch of salt
- ½ teaspoon crushed black pepper
- 2 slices of wheat bread

## Directions:

Take a pan and toss thin bagel in olive oil. After that in the same pan add oil and sauté the mushrooms, spinach leaves, avocado, red pepper, tomatoes, and add salt and pepper. Now cook the egg white. Take the bread slices and spread the bagel, eggs, and veggies on it in the form of layers. place the second slice on it and serve it.

**Nutrition:** Protein 13.1g, Fats 7.2g, Calories 278.6, Carbohydrates 42.1g, Fiber 4.0g.

# Chicken Caprese Sandwich

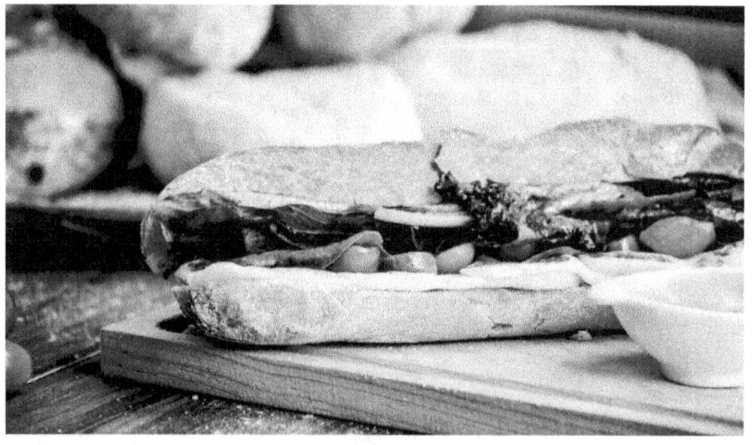

*Preparation time: 10 minutes I Cooking time: 10 minutes I Servings: 4*

**Ingredients:**

- ¼ cup prepared pesto
- 4 boneless chicken halves
- 8 basil leaves
- ¼ cup mayonnaise
- A pinch of salt and black pepper
- 1 sliced tomato
- 1 tablespoon olive oil
- 4 slices mozzarella cheese
- 4 slices of sandwich bread

**Directions:**

Grill the chicken with seasoning black pepper, salt, and olive oil. Grill the chicken for around 10 minutes. In a bowl mix the mayonnaise and pesto. Toast the bread slices and spread the mixed mayonnaise. Place the grilled chicken, leaves, tomatoes, and mozzarella cheese slice and serve it.

**Nutrition:** Protein 37g, fats 28g, Calories 542, Carbohydrates 33g, Fiber 1g.

# Slow-Cooker Split Pea Soup

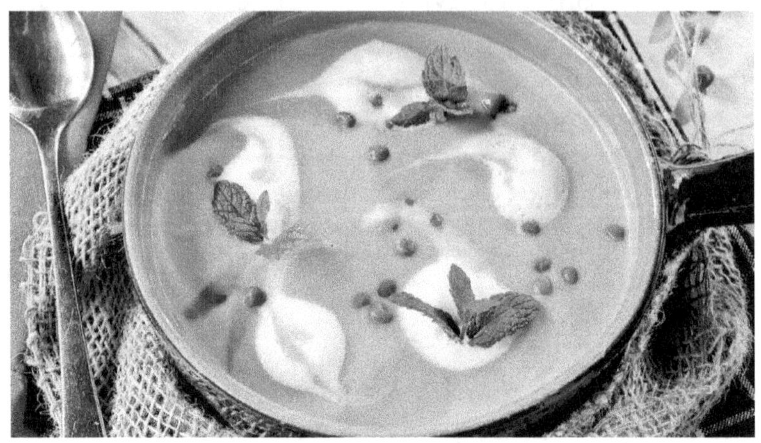

***Preparation time***: *10-15 minutes* | ***Cooking time***: *6-8 hours* | ***Servings***: *8*

## Ingredients:

- 2 cups fully cooked ham
- 1 chopped large onion
- 1 cup chopped carrots
- 3 minced garlic cloves
- 16 ounces dried split green peas
- 32 ounces chicken broth
- ½ teaspoon dried thyme
- ½ teaspoon crushed dried rosemary
- 2 cups of water

## Directions:

Take a slow cooker and add all the ingredients in it. Combine and mix them well. Cover the slow cooker and cook it on a medium flame for 6 to 8 hours. Cook until peas become soft. If you are using the uncooked ham it will take 10 hours to cook.

**Nutrition:** Protein 23g, Fats 2g, Calories 260, Sugar 7g, Carbohydrates 39g, Cholesterol 21mg.

# Cobb Egg Salad

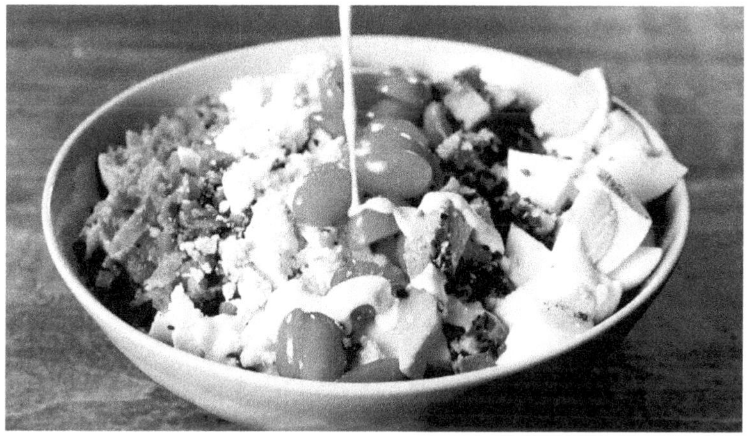

*Preparation time: 10 minutes I **Chilling time**: 5 minutes I **Servings**: 6*

## Ingredients:

- 3 tablespoons yogurt
- 8 hard-boiled eggs
- 3 tablespoons mayonnaise
- a pinch of crushed black pepper
- 2 tablespoons red wine vinegar
- a pinch of salt
- 8 strips of cooked bacon

- ½ cup finely grated cheese
- 1 thinly sliced avocado2 tablespoons crushed chives
- ½ cup cherry and tomatoes (for garnishing)

**Directions:**

Take a bowl and smashed the boiled eggs. Now add all the ingredients in the same bowl expect cherry and tomatoes. Mix all the ingredients until they combine well. Put it in the refrigerator for 5 minutes so that all the ingredients set well. Serve it after garnishing it with cherry and tomatoes.

**Nutrition:** Protein 13g, Fats 5g, Calories 235, Sugar 2g, Carbohydrates 9g, Cholesterol 195mg, Fiber 3g.

# Chicken Cheese Sandwich

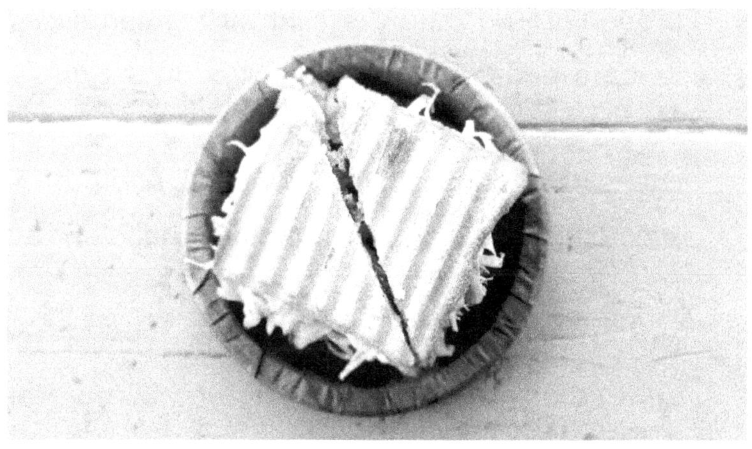

*Preparation time*: 10 minutes | *Cooking time*: 5 minutes | *Servings*: 4

## Ingredients:

- 4 tablespoons mayonnaise
- 1 ½ cups boiled and shredded chicken
- ½ cup thinly sliced cucumber
- ½ cup red capsicum
- ½ teaspoon crushed black pepper
- a pinch of salt
- ½ teaspoon crushed white pepper
- ½ cup sweet corn
- ½ cup finely grated cheese
- 2 tablespoons butter
- 8-10 slices of sandwich bread

## Directions:

Take a bowl and add all the ingredients in it except bread, butter, and cheese. Combine the ingredients properly. Now take the sandwich bread slices and cut its hard sides. Apply some butter on the one side of all the slices and toast them from both sides. Now add cheese and prepared mixture on it. And put the second slice on it. Cut it in the triangular shape and serve it.

**Nutrition:** Protein 8g, Fats 29g, Calories 369, Sugar 2g, Carbohydrates 16g, Cholesterol 35mg, Fiber 1g.

## Charred Shrimp And Avocado

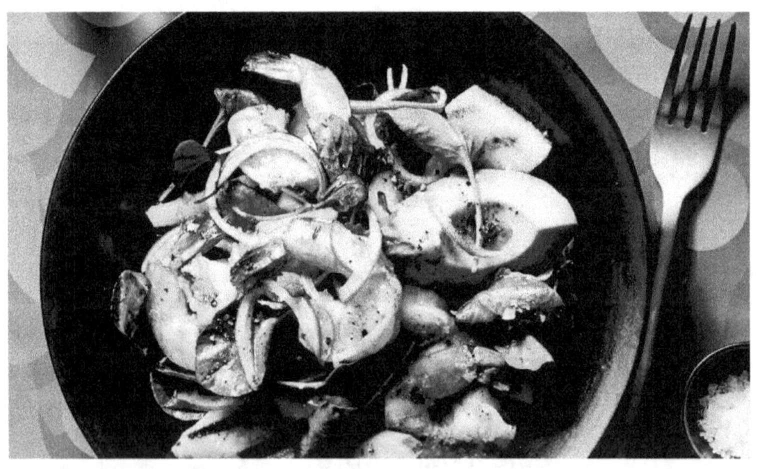

*Preparation time*: 10 minutes | *Cooking time*: 15 minutes | *Servings*: 4

**Ingredients:**

- 5 tablespoons olive oil
- 2 ½ lb. peeled large shrimp
- ½ teaspoon salt
- 1 cup peeled and cubed cut pineapple
- ½ cup thinly sliced onion
- 1 avocado
- 2 tablespoons lemon juice
- ½ cup finely peeled and cut cucumber
- ½ finely chopped upland watercress
- ½ teaspoon crushed
- black pepper

**Directions:**

Take a pan and toss shrimp in oil, salt, and pepper. Grill pineapple after brushing oil on both sides. Grill shrimp and pineapple for 3 minutes each side. Take another bowl and put all the remaining ingredients and mix them well. Now add the toasted shrimp and pineapple in it and present it.

**Nutrition:** Protein 35g, fats 23.5g, Calories 420, Carbohydrates 20g, Fiber 4g.

# Grilled Steak Tortilla

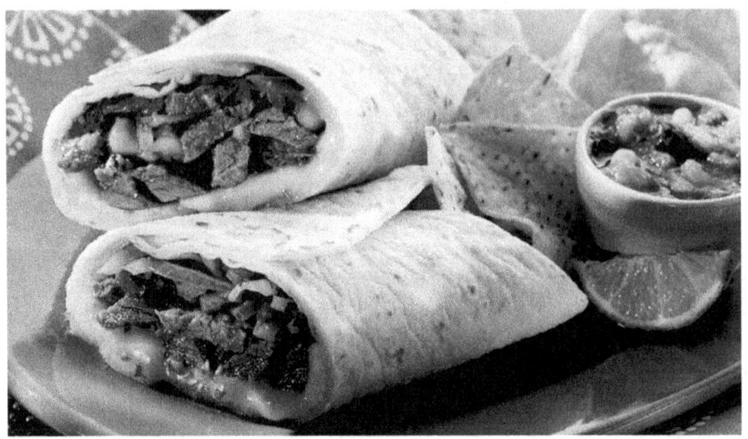

***Preparation time***: *10 minutes* / ***Cooking time***: *20 minutes* / ***Servings***: *4*

## Ingredients:

- 1 cup cubed cut tomatoes
- 1 cup brisket
- 1 teaspoon red chili powder
- 2 sliced cut spring onions
- 1 cup coriander
- 2 tablespoons lemon juice
- 1 sliced cut jalapeno
- 1 bunch of rocket
- 4 quarter cut flour tortillas
- 1 teaspoon salt

## Directions:

Grill the brisket with salt and paper for around 5 minutes. Mix the rest of the ingredients except tortillas.

Cut the slices of the grilled brisket and combine it in the mixture. Serve it with flour tortillas.

**Nutrition:** Protein 41g, fats 5g, Calories 420, Carbohydrates 9g, Fiber 3g.

## One-Pot Beef With Broccoli

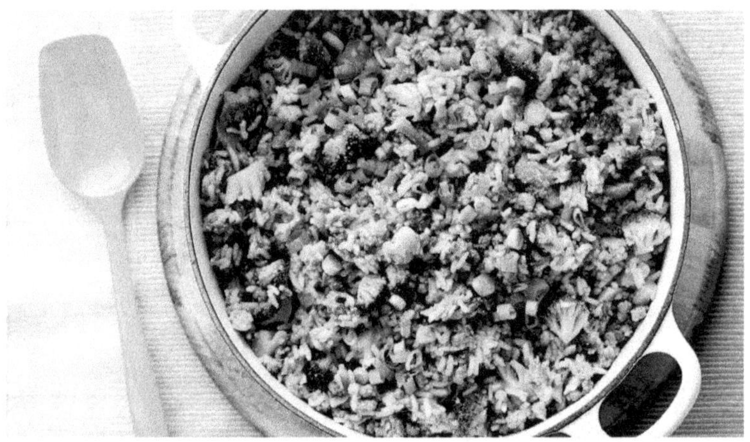

***Preparation time****: 10 minutes I **Cooking time***: *10 minutes I **Servings***: 5*

### Ingredients:

- 1½ cups chopped and cooked broccoli
- 1lb minced beef
- 3 cups cooked cold white rice
- 1 bunch chopped green onion
- ½ cup diced chopped white onion
- 1 cup teriyaki marinade and sauce
- A pinch of salt

**Directions:**

Take a nonstick pan with oil and cook beef over medium flame. Add salt in it and stir it continuously. Cook it for 5 to 7 minutes. Add onions in it and cook for one minute now add rice and teriyaki and sauce and cook for 2 minutes. Add broccoli in it and mix well. its ready to present.

**Nutrition:** Protein 28g, Fats 35g, Calories 460, Carbohydrates 7g, Fiber 1g.

# Sheet Pan Sausages & Veggies

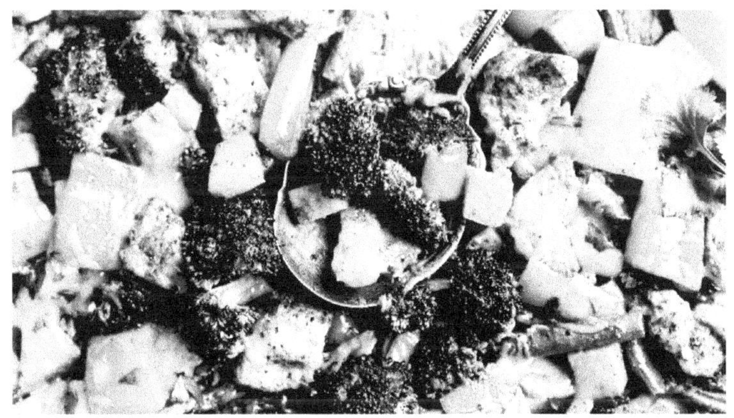

*Preparation time:  10 minutes I **Cooking time:  20 minutes I Servings: 4***

**Ingredients:**

- 1 diced red bell pepper
- 16 ounces smoked sausage

- 1 cup cubed radish
- ½ minced onion
- 1 teaspoon Italian seasoning
- 1 teaspoon salt
- 1 tablespoon halved parsley
- ½ teaspoon cracked pepper
- 2 tablespoons avocado oil
- 12 ounces florets broccoli

**Directions:**

Prepare a baking dish with liner and preheat the oven at 400F. Take a bowl and add all the ingredients except broccoli in it and mix them well. On the prepared baking dish spread the mixture in the single layer. Bake it for around 20 minutes in the preheated oven. Stir it once while baking. Sprinkle parsley on it and serve.

**Nutrition:** Protein 16g, Fats 39g, Calories 460, Carbohydrates 11g, Fiber 4g.

# Loaded Sheet Pan Nachos

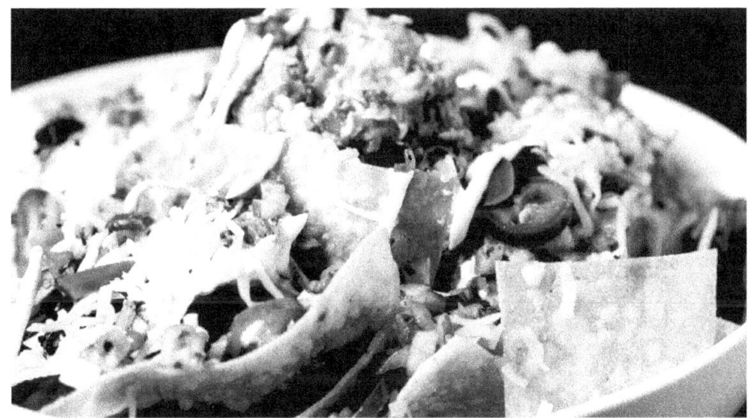

*Preparation time*:  15 minutes I *Cooking time*:  10 minutes I *Servings*: 8

**Ingredients:**

- 1 pound ground beef
- 12 ounces tortilla chips
- 1 tablespoon olive oil
- 2 chopped garlic cloves
- 1.25-ounce taco seasoning
- 1 cup roasted corn kernels
- 1 cup shredded cheddar cheese
- ½ cup grated Jack cheese
- 2 tablespoons sour cream
- 2 tablespoons chopped cilantro leaves
- 1 diced tomato
- 1 thinly sliced jalapeno

**Directions:**

Preheat the oven at 400F and prepare a baking dish with a baking sheet. Take a skillet with olive oil over the medium flame. Cook beef with garlic and cook it for 5 minutes. Add taco seasoning o it. In the baking dish place the chips in a single layer and spread beef mixture on it. Add beans, cheese, and corn on it and bake for 5 minutes. Topped it with remaining ingredients and serve it immediately.

**Nutrition:** Protein 24.3g, Fats 25.8g, Calories 493, Carbohydrates 44.1g, Fiber 7g.

# Lemon & Garlic Salmon With Asparagus

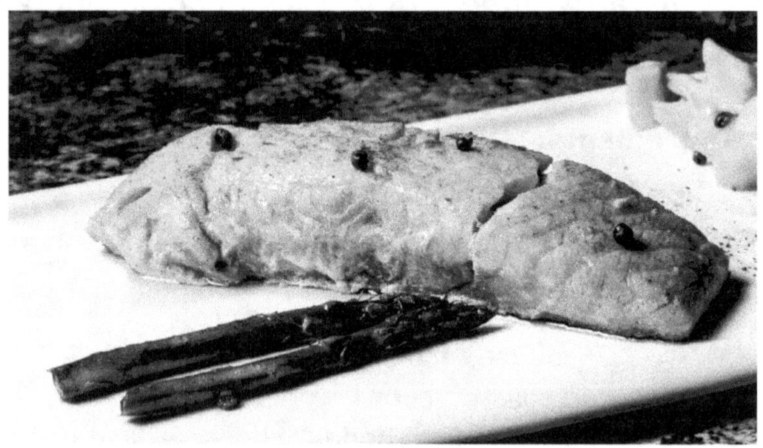

*Preparation time*:  *05 minutes* I ***Cooking time***:  *10 minutes* I **Servings**: *3*

## Ingredients:

- 1 tablespoon salted butter
- 2 chopped garlic cloves
- 1 tablespoon olive oil
- 1 trimmed bunch of asparagus
- 1 pound fillet cut salmon

- ½ tablespoon lemon juice
- ½ teaspoon salt and black pepper

**Directions:**

Heat the butter and olive oil in a skillet. Add asparagus and salmon in it and season with pepper and salt. Cook it for around 3 to 4 minutes on each side. Add garlic and lemon juice and cook for 1 to 2 minutes more. Convert it into the serving dish and serve.

**Nutrition:** Protein 32.8g, Fats 28.8g, Calories 409, Carbohydrates 4.6g, Cholesterol 93.3mg.

# Slow Cooker BBQ Chicken

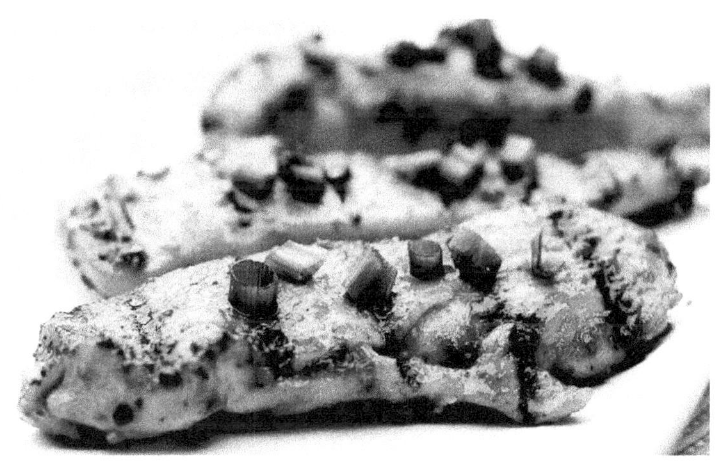

*Preparation time:* *5 minutes I* ***Cooking time:*** *4 hours I* ***Servings:*** *4*

## Ingredients:

- 4 boneless chicken breasts
- ½ chopped onion
- 1 tablespoon soy sauce
- 1½ cups BBQ sauce
- 1 tablespoon olive oil
- 2 tablespoons brown sugar

## Directions:

In a slow cooker add all the ingredients and mix them well. Coat the chicken in sauce mixture thoroughly. Cover and cook it on medium heat for 4 hours. Now remove the chicken in a trey and shred it with the help of forks. Serve it with some BBQ sauce topping.

**Nutrition:** Protein 23.1g, Fats 2.8g, Calories 364, Carbohydrates 59.9g.

# Crispy Cauliflower Tacos

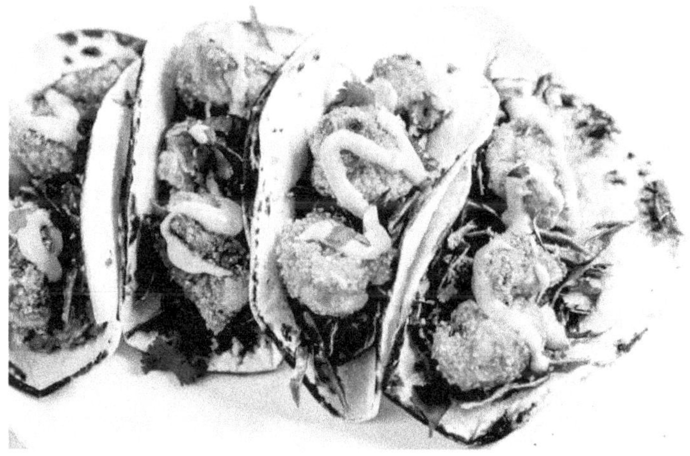

*Preparation time*: 15 minutes | *Cooking time*: 30 minutes | *Servings*: 12


## Ingredients:

- ¾ cup chickpea flour
- ¾ cup almond milk
- 3 tablespoons taco seasoning
- 1 ½ cup cornmeal
- 1 cauliflower
- 3 cups grated cabbage
- 12 sugar free tortillas
- 2 tablespoons yeast
- ½ teaspoon salt and pepper


## Directions:

Cut the cauliflower in thick pieces. Take a bowl and mix the flour and almond milk in it and leave it for few minutes. In another bowl mix yeast, taco, salt and pepper, and cornmeal. Now dip each piece of cauliflower in the flour and yeast mixture one by one. Set this cauliflower on the baking sheet and put it in the preheated oven with 400F temperature for 25 to 30 minutes. Now place the pieces of backed cauliflower in the tortillas and add cabbage on it. And it's ready to serve.

**Nutrition:** Protein 10g, Fats 5g, Calories 230, Carbohydrates 37g, Fiber 9g.

# Chicken Scampi Pasta

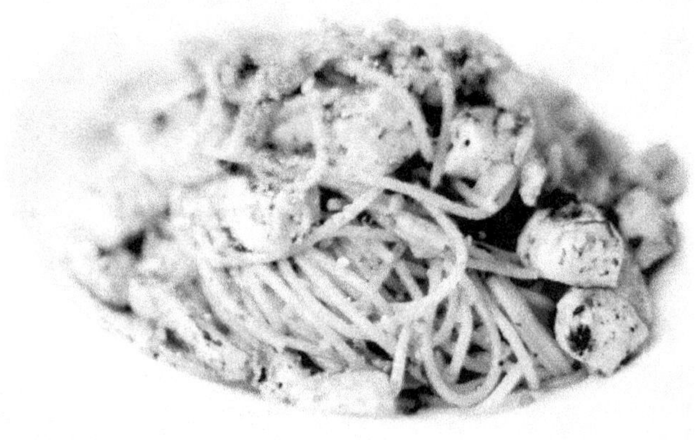

*Preparation time:* *10 minutes I* **Cooking time**: *10 minutes I* **Servings**: *6*

## Ingredients:

- 2 cups boiled pasta
- 3 sliced chicken breasts
- 1 finely sliced bell pepper

- 1 tablespoon Italian seasoning
- ½ sliced cut onion
- 2 cups chicken broth
- 1 minced garlic clove
- ½ teaspoon salt
- ½ teaspoon black pepper
- 1 cup sheared cheese

**Directions:**

Take a skillet and place the sliced chicken breast in it. Cook it over medium-high flame until its color started to change. Add onion and bell peppers in it and cook for more 2 to 3 minutes. Add broth in it and when it starts simmering reduce the heat and cover it with the lid. Take a dish with boiled pasta and add cooked chicken and cheese on it. Sprinkle salt and pepper on it and serve it immediately.

**Nutrition:** Protein 29g, fats 7g, Calories 435, Carbohydrates 60g, Fiber 3g.

# Chicken Steak With Stuffed Potatoes

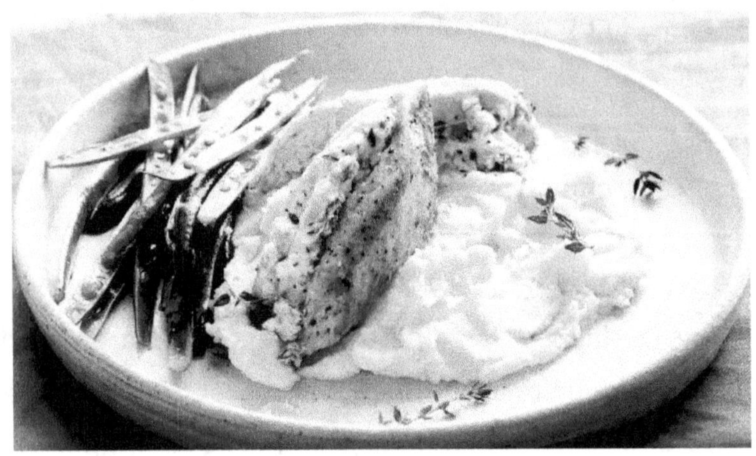

***Preparation time****: 25 minutes I **Cooking time***: 45 minutes I **Servings***: 4*

## Ingredients:

- 2 potatoes
- 4 chicken breasts
- ½ teaspoon salt
- 1 tablespoon olive oil
- ½ teaspoon crushed black pepper
- 1 tablespoon butter
- 1 minced garlic clove
- ½ teaspoon salt
- ½ tablespoon lemon juice
- 2 tablespoon ginger and garlic paste
- ½ tablespoon red chilly
- ¼ teaspoon cinnamon powder

## Directions:

Peel and cut the potatoes. Boil them on a medium flame for around 20 minutes. Mash these boiled potatoes and mix milk, butter, salt, and black pepper in it. Put it aside. Take the chicken breasts and make a pocket in it by cutting it from the middle. Take a bowl add garlic and ginger paste, lemon juice, red pepper, salt, cinnamon powder in it and mix it well. Marinate the chicken with the mixture and leave it for at least 15 minutes. Stuffed the potato mixture in the chicken breast. Now take a grill pan and cook the chicken stakes for at least 10 minutes. Then low down the flame and cover the pan and cook for more 5 minutes. Take out on the serving plate and serve it.

**Nutrition:** Protein 19g, Fats 12g, Calories 370, Carbohydrates 69g, Fiber 7g.

## Buffalo Chicken Enchiladas

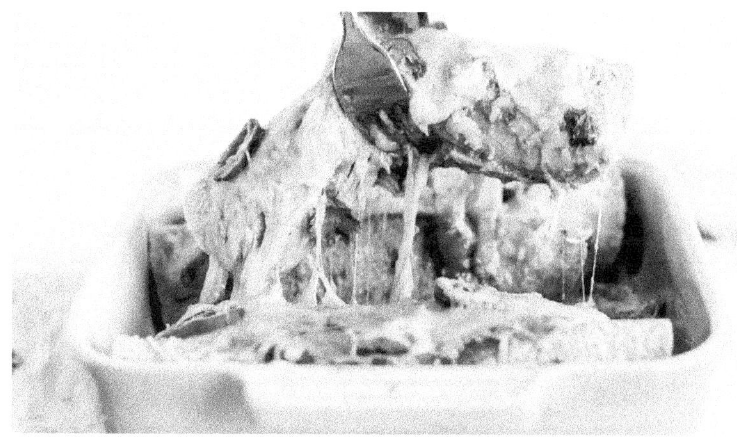

***Preparation time**: 10 minutes | **Cooking time**: 20 minutes | **Servings**: 4*

## Ingredients:

- ½ teaspoon seasoning
- 1 boiled and shredded chicken breast
- ½ cup buffalo sauce
- ½ cup enchilada sauce
- ½ cup cubed cut tomatoes
- 5 flour tortillas
- 1 cup shredded cheese
- ½ teaspoon crushed green chilies

## Directions:

Prepare the baking dish with a baking sheet and add the half enchilada sauce in it. Preheat the oven at the 350F temperature. Take a bowl and mix the chicken, buffalo sauce, remaining enchilada sauce, tomatoes and green chilly in it and combine well. Take the tortillas and pour chicken mixture in its middle and add cheese on its top. Now fold it from two sides on the filling portion. Set them in the baking dish and add cheese and sauces on its top. Now bake it in the preheated oven for around 20 minutes.

**Nutrition:** Protein 15g, Fats 3g, Calories 191, Carbohydrates 22g, Fiber 1g, Cholesterol 36mg.

# Hot Sausages Cast-Iron Skillet Pan Pizza

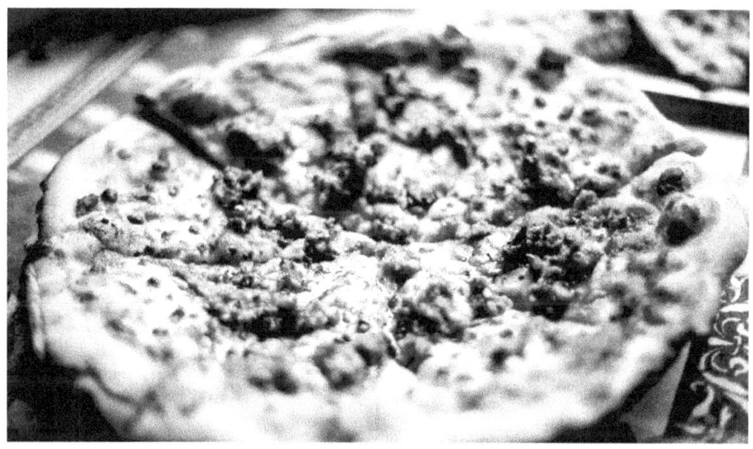

*Preparation time*:  15 minutes I ***Cooking time***:  30 minutes I ***Servings***: 4

## Ingredients:

- 2 tablespoons tomato paste
- 1 cup cubed tomatoes
- A pinch of salt and black pepper
- a pinch of sugar
- ¼ teaspoon oregano
- 1 minced garlic clove
- 6-7 leaves of basil
- 1 pound pizza dough
- ¼ cup oil
- ½ pound diced hot sausage
- 3 cups grated cheese

**Directions:**

In a blender add tomato paste, garlic, oregano, basil, sugar, and salt and blend it well. Take a greased skillet and stretch the dough in the even round shape. Take a pan with oil and cook the sausages until it changes its color. Now take the pan and set the pizza dough in it. Now brush oil on the dough and add the blended sauce on it. Add cooked sausages, and cheese. Now cook it on the medium-low flame for around 3 minutes. Transfer it from skillet to the baking dish. And bake it in the preheated oven at the 475F temperature for around 15 minutes.

**Nutrition:** Protein 36g, Fats 3g, Calories 390, Carbohydrates 29g, Fiber 5g.

# Delicious Snacks Recipes

## Potato Lollipop

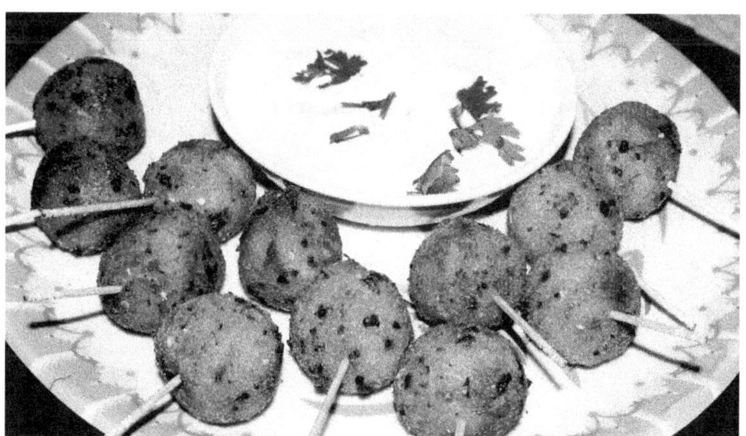

**Preparation time**: *15 minutes* I **Cooking time**: *15 minutes* I **Servings**: *3*

### Ingredients:

- 2 large boiled and peeled potatoes
- 2 chopped green chilies
- 2 slices of bread
- 1 boiled and peeled carrot
- ½ teaspoon ginger paste
- 2 teaspoons corn flour
- ½ teaspoon cumin powder
- 2 cups oil
- ½ teaspoon salt

- ½ teaspoon chaat masala powder

**Directions:**

In a bowl mash the boiled potatoes and add carrots, ginger, green chilies, chaat masala, cumin powder, and salt in it and mix all the ingredients properly. Soak the slices of bread in water for 3 minutes and squeeze the water properly. Add in the potato mixture and add corn flour too. Mix all the ingredients and make small balls with this dough. Shallow fry these balls properly and insert a lollipop stick in it and serve.

**Nutrition:** Protein 2g, Fats 3g, Calories 187, Carbohydrates 12g, Fiber 1g, Cholesterol 1mg.

# Potato Cheese Balls

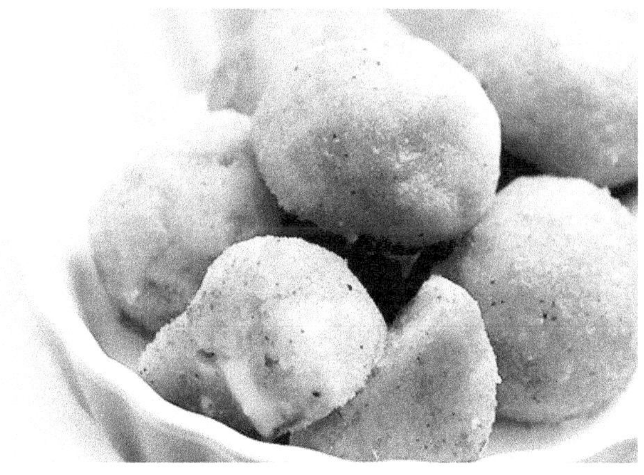

*Preparation time*:  *15 minutes* | ***Cooking time***:  *10 minutes* | ***Servings***: *10*

## Ingredients:

- 2 ½ cups boiled mashed potatoes
- ½ cup cheddar cheese
- ½ teaspoon salt
- ½ teaspoon white pepper
- 1 cup breadcrumbs
- 2 lightly beaten eggs
- 1 cup flour
- 1 cup vegetable oil

## Directions:

Take a bowl and add mashed potatoes, salt, and white pepper mix it well. Now make balls of it by adding small cheese slice in its middle. Now coat it in the flour, egg, and breadcrumbs in a sequence. Shallow fry them in the vegetable oil on the medium heat. Serve them immediately.

**Nutrition:** Fats 4g, Calories 110, Carbohydrates 15g, Cholesterol 24mg.

# Crispy Pepperoni Chips

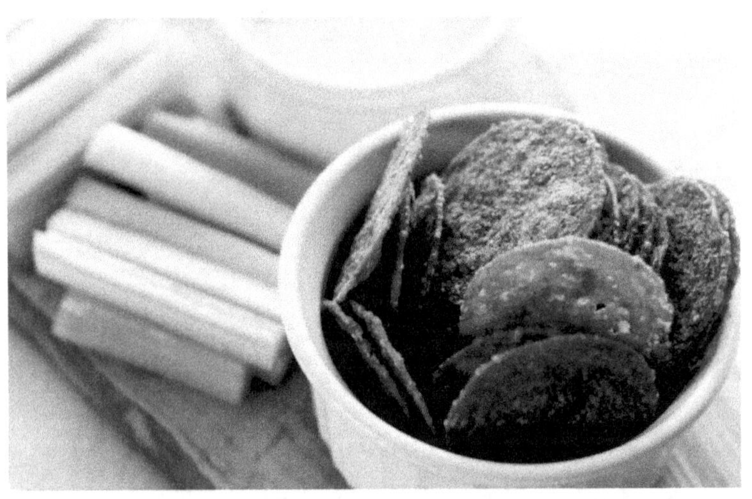

*Preparation time*:  *05 minutes I* ***Cooking time***:  *15 minutes I **Servings**: 4*

**Ingredients:**
- 6 ounces thinly sliced pepperoni

**Directions:**

Preheat the oven at the 425 degrees F temperature. Prepare a baking dish with liner. Spread the pepperoni slices on baking dish in a single layer. Bake it in the preheated oven for around 10 minutes. Take out the pan from the oven and with the help of a soaking sheet or towel soak the excess grease from the pepperoni. Put the pan in the oven again for around 4 to 5 minutes until pepperoni slices become crispy.

**Nutrition:** Fats 14g, Calories 150, Carbohydrates 1g, Cholesterol 30mg, Protein 5g

# Candied Almonds

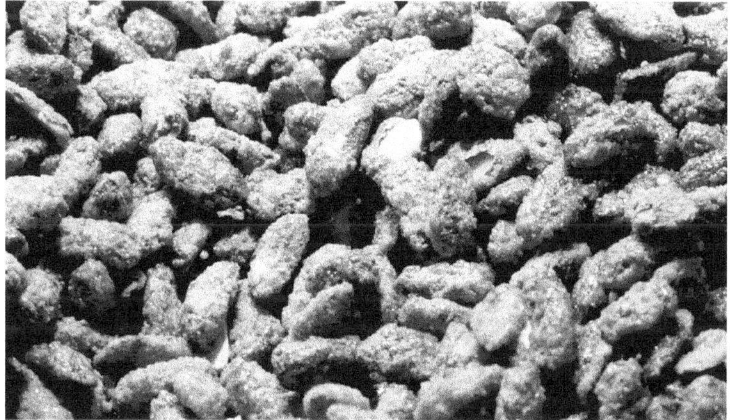

*Preparation time*: *05 minutes* | *Cooking time*: *15 minutes* | *Servings*: *08*

**Ingredients:**

- 1 cup white sugar
- ½ cup water
- 2 cups almonds
- 1 tablespoon ground cinnamon

**Directions:**

In a pan add water, cinnamon, and sugar and put it on the medium flame. When it starts boiling add almonds in it. Cook it until the water evaporates and the mixture transformed in the form of a syrup or coating around the almonds. Now dish out the coated almond and leave them to cool for 15 minutes. Now it is ready to present.

**Nutrition:** Fats 18g, Calories 304, Carbohydrates 32.7g, Protein 7.6g.

# Wheat Crackers

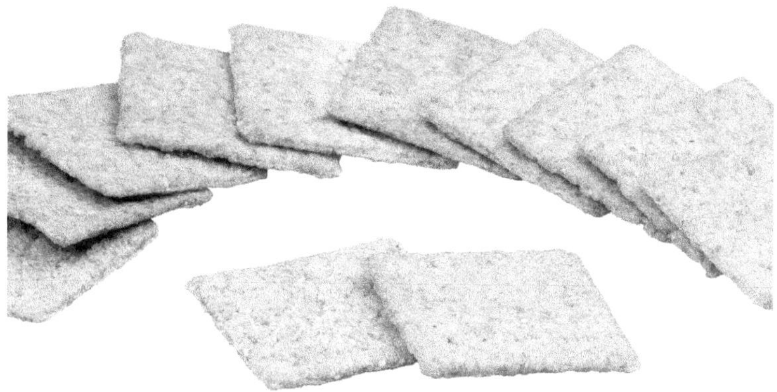

***Preparation time****:  10 minutes I **Cooking time***: 20 minutes I ***Servings***: 32

## Ingredients:

- 1 ½ cups all-purpose flour
- 1 ¾ cups whole wheat flour
- 1/3 cup vegetable oil
- ¾ teaspoon salt
- 1 cup of water

## Directions:

In a bowl add all the ingredients and mix them until it gets the form of a dough. Preheat the oven at 350F temperature. Roll out the prepared dough on a light surface with flour in a thinner layer. It should be thinner than 1/8 inch. Now place it in the ungreased baking dish. With the help of knife mark squares and with the help of fork prick each piece of cracker. Sprinkle a pinch of salt and bake it for 20 minutes or until it becomes crispy.

**Nutrition:** Fats 2.5g, Calories 64, Carbohydrates 9.2g, Protein 1.5g.

# Cranberry Nut Granola Bar

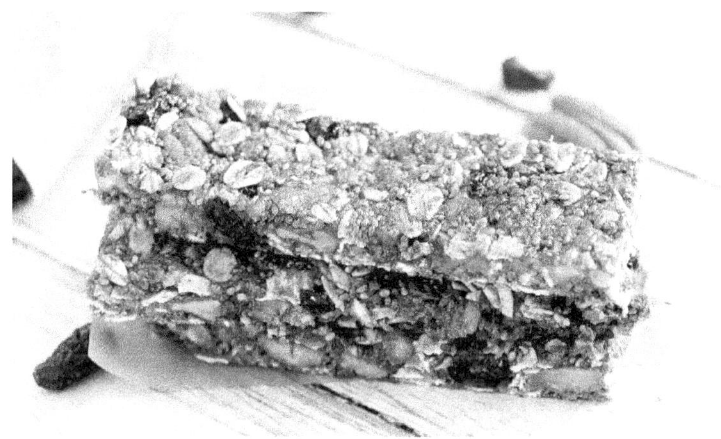

**Preparation time**: *10 minutes* | **Cooking time**: *20 minutes* | **Servings**: *24*

## Ingredients:

- ½ cup slivered almonds
- 1 cup mix nuts
- 2 cups oats
- ½ cup hulled pumpkin seeds
- 1 cup condensed milk
- 1 cup cranberries

## Directions:

In a mixing bowl mix all the ingredients thoroughly. Preheat the oven at the temperature of 350F. Prepare a baking dish with greased baking liner on all sides. Spread it into the baking dish in a thick layer evenly. Bake it in for around 20 to 25 minutes. Let it be cool for

5 minutes and cut it in the form of bars with a sharp knife and serve it.

**Nutrition:** Fats 7.5g, Calories 169, Carbohydrates 22.3g, Protein 4.8g.

# Bacon Avocado Fries

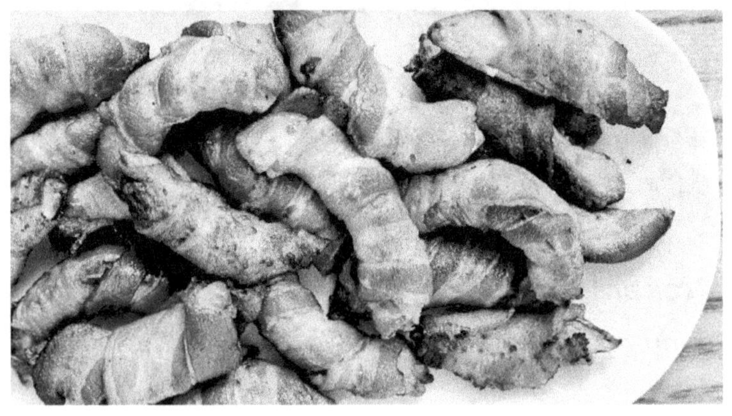

*Preparation time:*  *10 minutes* I ***Chilling time:***  *15 minutes* I ***Servings****: 20*

## Ingredients:

- 3 thinly sliced avocados
- 20 thin strips bacon
- ¼ cup ranch dressing (optional)

## Directions:

Prepare a baking dish with a greased baking sheet. Set the oven at 425F temperature to preheat. Take a thin slice of avocado and wrap it in the bacon slice properly. Wrap all the avocado slices in the bacon slices. Place them in the prepared baking dish and bake for around 15 minutes or until it becomes crispy. Now pour ranch dressing on it if you want to.

**Nutrition:** Fats 65.9g, Calories 693, Carbohydrates 10.9g, Protein 16.3g.

# Jalapeno Popper Crisps

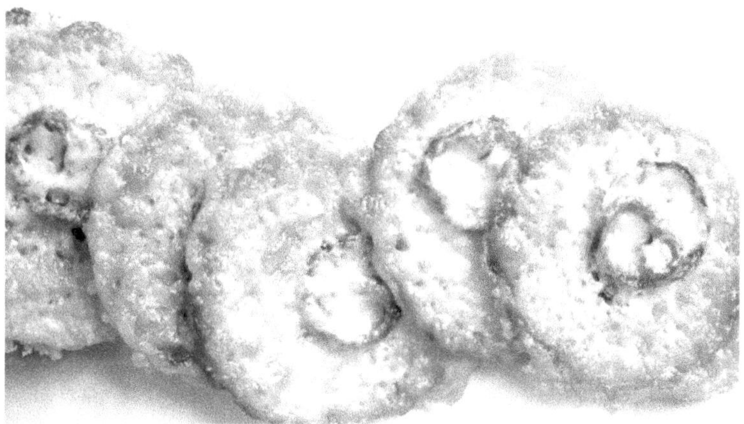

*Preparation time:  10 minutes I **Cooking time**:  15 minutes I **Servings**: 8*

## Ingredients:

- 1 cup grated parmesan
- ½ cup grated cheddar cheese
- ½ teaspoon crushed black pepper
- 1 thinly sliced jalapeno

- 4 slices bacon

**Directions:**

Preheat the oven at the 375F. In a nonstick skillet cook the bacon for around 8 minutes. Drain the grease with the help of a paper towel and chop it. In the lined baking dish carefully spread 1 tablespoon parmesan. Add 1 tablespoon cheddar cheese on its top and add a jalapeno slice on it. Now carefully pats with and sprinkle pepper on it. Make such small circles with the same process in the whole tray with some distance. Bake it for 12 minutes and serve it when it slightly cooled down.

**Nutrition:** Fats 12g, Calories 153, Cholesterol 39mg, Protein 9g.

# Peanut Butter Protein Balls

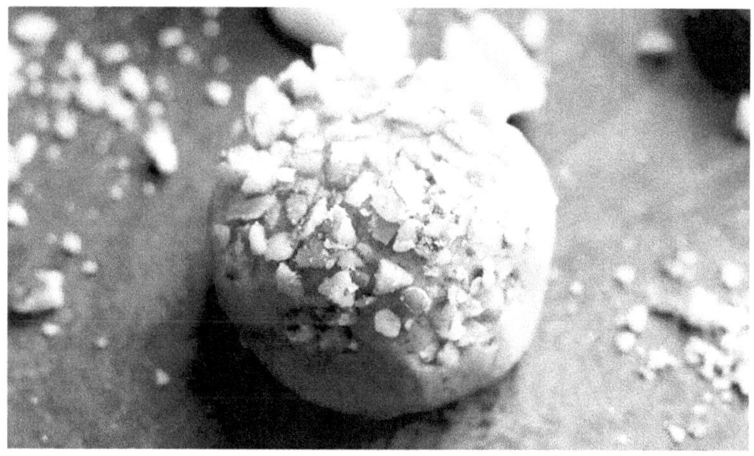

***Preparation time****:   10 minutes |* ***Chilling time****:   15 minutes |* ***Servings****: 15*

## Ingredients:

- 1 cup unsalted peanut butter
- ½ teaspoon vanilla extract
- 2 teaspoon brown sugar
- 1½ scoops vanilla protein powder
- 20 unsalted raw peanuts
- 1 teaspoon cinnamon

## Directions:

Blend the raw peanuts in a blunder and when they become crumbly transfer it to a plate. Take a bowl and add all the ingredients except blended peanuts. Mix them properly. Make the balls with the batter and roll them in the peanut crumble. Set them in a dish and refrigerate it for 15 minutes.

**Nutrition:** Fats 9.6g, Calories 126, Carbohydrates 4.7g, Protein 7.6g, Sugar 0.7g.

# Veggies Cheese Rolls

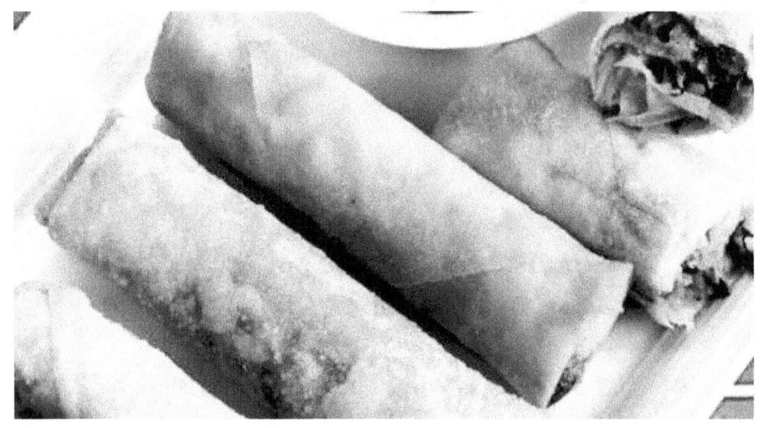

*Preparation time*: *15 minutes* I *Cooking time*: *15 minutes* I *Servings*: *4*

## Ingredients:

- 1 chopped onion
- 1 chopped tomato
- 1 cup shattered cabbage
- 3 chopped florets broccoli
- 4 tortillas
- ¼ cup coriander leaves
- 2 cups shattered cheese

- 1 beaten egg

**Directions:**

In a pan sauté the onion, tomato, cabbage, broccoli, coriander leaves for 2 to 3 minutes. In the end, add cheese on it and remove it from the stove. Mix all the ingredients well. Now take the tortillas and add some prepared mixture in it and roll it nicely. Close its sides with beaten egg. Place it in the prepared baking tray with the baking paper. Bake it in the preheated oven with 180C temperature for 20 minutes.

**Nutrition:** Fats 26g, Calories 391, Carbohydrates 27g, Protein 12g, Sugar 6g.

# Strawberry Smoothie

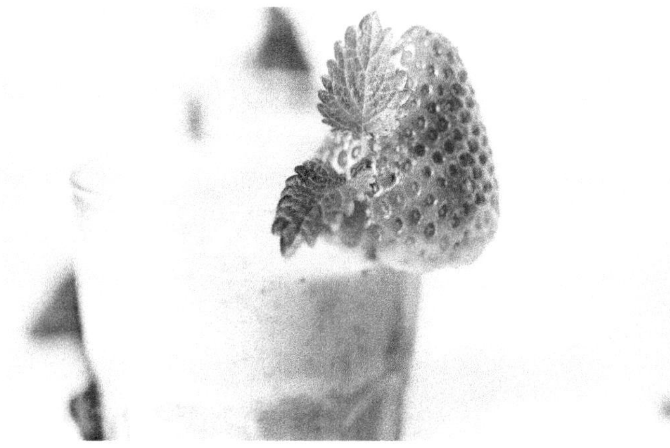

*Preparation time: 5 minutes | **Chilling time**: 30 minutes | **Servings**: 2*

## Ingredients:

- 1 cup low-fat milk
- 1 cup frozen strawberries
- 1 tablespoon peanut butter
- 1 teaspoon vanilla extract
- ¼ cup low-fat yogurt

## Directions:

Take a high power blender. Put all the ingredients including butter, milk, yogurt, honey, vanilla extract, and strawberries in the blender and blend it until every ingredient merged well. Put it in the glass and leave it to chill for 30 minutes. You can take it immediately as well by adding ice cubes in it.

**Nutrition:** Protein 6g, Fats 3g, Calories 130, Carbohydrates 15g, Fiber 3g, Cholesterol 1mg.

# Caramel Popcorn

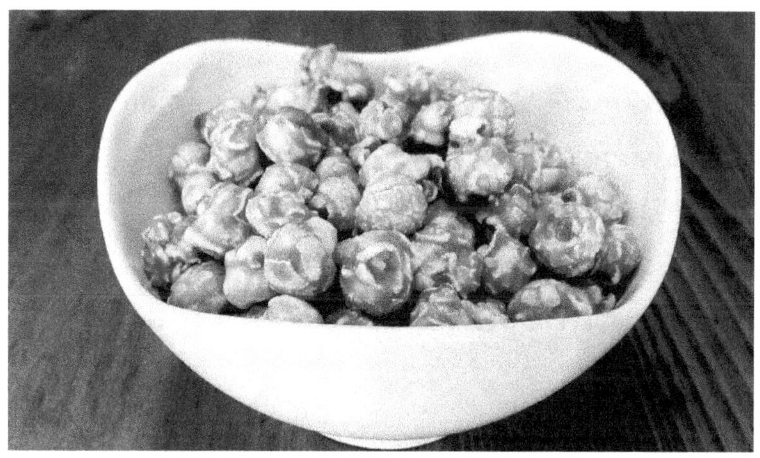

***Preparation time***: *10 minutes* I ***Cooking time***: *10 minutes* I ***Servings***: *10*

## Ingredients:

- 1 cup butter
- 10 cups popped popcorns
- ½ teaspoon salt
- 2 teaspoons vanilla
- 1 cup brown sugar
- ½ teaspoon baking soda

## Directions:

Salt the popped popcorns and set aside. Now take a pan and melt the butter on the medium flame. Add sugar in it and stir it thoroughly and continuously. When it starts boiling leave it on the medium flame for the 5 minutes. Put vanilla in it and mix it well and keep it on the stove for 4 minutes. Now add baking soda in it and cook for another minute. Now pour this mixture on the popcorns and mix it gently. Leave it for some time to keep it cool.

**Nutrition:** Fats 10g, Calories 245, Carbohydrates 38g, Cholesterol 20mg.

# Chocolate Chip Cookies

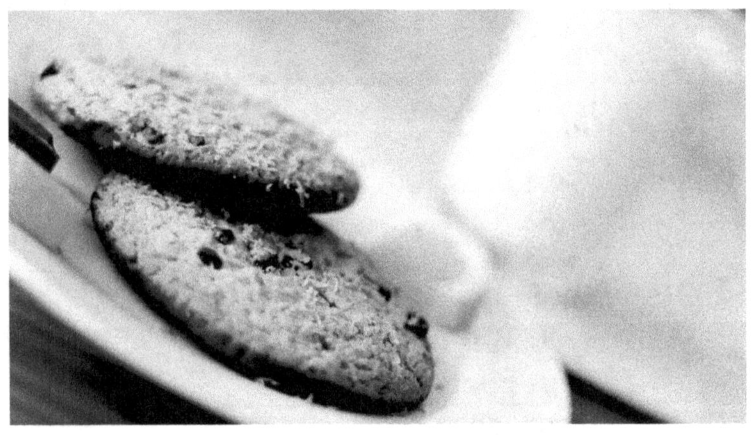

*Preparation time:*  *10 minutes I* ***Cooking time****:  8 minutes I* ***Servings****: 12*

## Ingredients:

- 1 cup brown sugar
- 1 cup butter
- 2 teaspoons vanilla extract
- 1 cup white sugar
- 3 cups flour
- 2 large eggs
- 1 teaspoon baking soda
- 1 teaspoon salt

- 2 cups chocolate chips

**Directions:**

Take a bowl and mix flour, salt, baking powder, and baking soda and set it aside. Add butter and sugar and beat it well. Now add eggs and vanilla in it and beat it well. Mix it in the dry ingredients until it merged well. Add chocolate chips in it. Take a baking dish with baking sheet. Use the scope for making the cookies. Put it in the 375 degrees F preheated oven. And cook it for around 8 to 10 minutes. After 2 minutes remove it in the serving plate.

**Nutrition:** Fats 12.6g, Calories 263, Carbohydrates 41g, Cholesterol 31.6mg, Protein 2.7g, Sugar 25.5g.

# Granola Bars

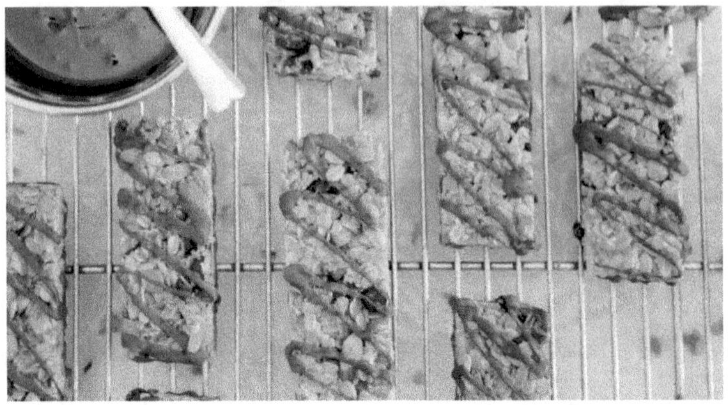

***Preparation time***:  *25 minutes* | ***Cooking time***:  *25 minutes* | ***Servings***: *18*

## Ingredients:

- 1/3 cup honey
- 2 tablespoons brown sugar
- 6 tablespoons melted butter
- 2 tablespoons maple syrup
- ¼ teaspoon salt
- 1 teaspoon cinnamon powder
- ½ cup shredded coconut
- 3 cups rolled oats
- ½ cup crushed almonds
- 1 ½ cups melted dark chocolate

## Directions:

Set the baking tray with baking line and preheat the oven at the 350 degrees F. place a pan on the low medium flame and add honey, butter, cinnamon, maple syrup, and brown sugar. Let it simmer and remove it from the stove when all the ingredients merged well. Now put all the remaining ingredients in it and mix it well. Pour it in the baking tray in an even layer. Bake it in the preheated oven for around 25 to 30 minutes. And cut it in the form of bars.

**Nutrition:** Fats 13g, Calories 199, Carbohydrates 21g, Cholesterol 10mg, Protein 2g, Sugar 10g.

# Nutella Sandwich

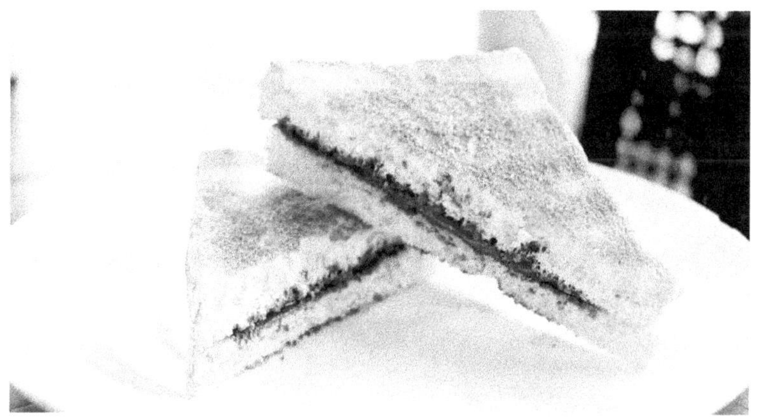

*Preparation time:  5 minutes | **Cooking time**:  5 minutes | **Servings**: 3*

## Ingredients:

- 6 slices of sandwich bread
- 1 teaspoon butter
- ¾ cup Nutella

## Directions:

Take the slices of bread and cut its hard sides. Now apply butter on both sides and grill it for around a minute on each side or until its color changed into golden. Now take the Nutella and apply it on the bread slices. Cut it in the triangular shape and present it. If you are banana lover, you can also use mashed banana in its filling besides Nutella.

**Nutrition:** Fats 10g, Calories 308, Carbohydrates 46g, Cholesterol 0mg, Protein 6.7g, Sugar 19g.

# Oreo Truffles

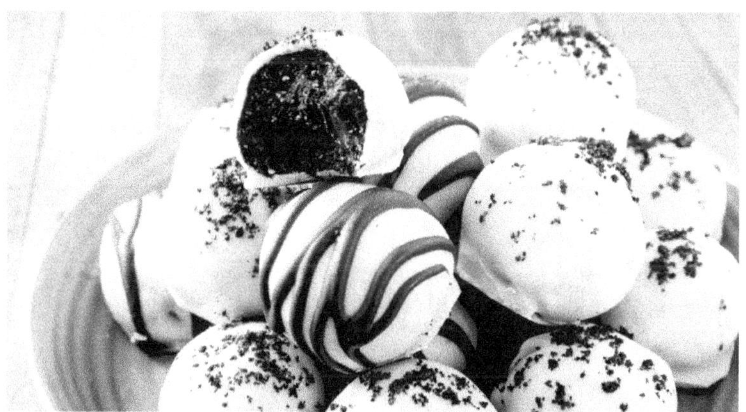

**Preparation time**: *05 minutes* I **Chilling time**: *1 hour* I **Servings**: *12*

## Ingredients:

- 8 oz. softened cream cheese
- 14 oz. Oreos
- 2 cups melted white chocolate
- 1 teaspoon vanilla extract
- ½ cup melted the dark chocolate

## Directions:

In a blender blend the Oreo cookies to transform it in crumbs. In a bowl mix all the ingredients leaving half white chocolate. Now make small balls of this batter and dip it in the remaining melted white chocolate. Refrigerate it for an hour and serve it.

**Nutrition:** Fats 6g, Calories 118, Carbohydrates 13g, Protein 1g.

# Chocolate Covered Cake Balls

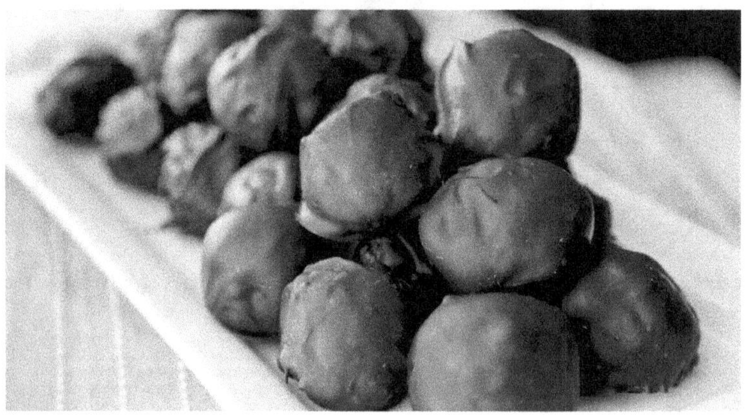

*Preparation time: 10 minutes I Chilling time: 1 hour 3' I Servings: 25*

**Ingredients:**

- 18.25 chocolate cake fudge
- 16 oz. prepared chocolate frosting
- 16 oz. dipping chocolate

**Directions:**

Put the fudge cake into a bowl and crumbled it thoroughly. Add the chocolate frosting in it and mix it well. Make the small balls of this batter and refrigerate it for 20 minutes. Take the balls out and dip them in the dipping chocolate one by one. Now put it back in the refrigerator for one hour and serve it.

**Nutrition:** Fats 6g, Calories 146, Carbohydrates 22g, sugar 17g.

# Pumpkin Cake Roll

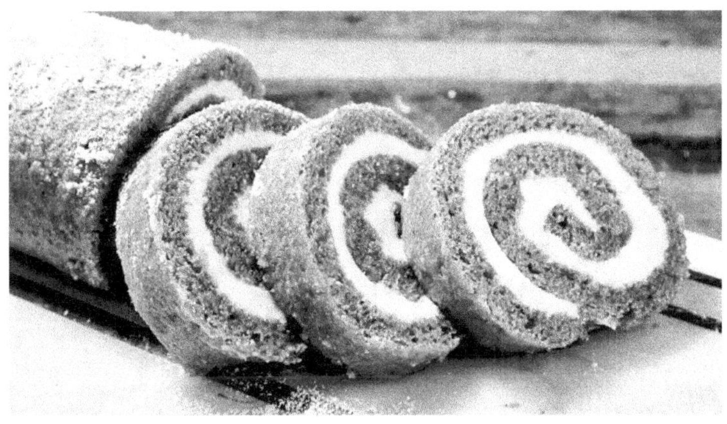

*Preparation time:* 20 minutes / *Cooking time:* 15 minutes / *Servings:* 10

**Ingredients:**
- 1 cup sugar

- 3 eggs
- ½ teaspoon crushed cinnamon
- 1 teaspoon baking soda
- ¾ cup flour
- 2/3 cup canned pumpkin
- 1 pinch salt
- 2 tablespoons softened butter
- 8 ounces softened cream cheese
- ¾ teaspoon vanilla extract

**Directions:**

Prepare a baking tray with greased liner. In a bowl beat eggs, then add ½ cup sugar, baking soda, cinnamon, flour, pumpkin, and salt. Beat and mix all the ingredients thoroughly. In the prepared pan spread the mixture evenly in a layer. Bake it at the 375 degrees preheated oven for 12 minutes. Put the baked cake on the sugar-dusted kitchen towel and roll the cake. Now in a bowl mix the butter, remaining sugar, vanilla extract, and cream cheese. Mix all the ingredients well and spread it in the cake after opening up and again roll it. Cut it into the pieces and serve.

**Nutrition:** Fats 12.4g, Calories 228, Carbohydrates 27g, Protein 3.9g, Cholesterol 54mg.

# Peanut Butter No-Bake Cookies

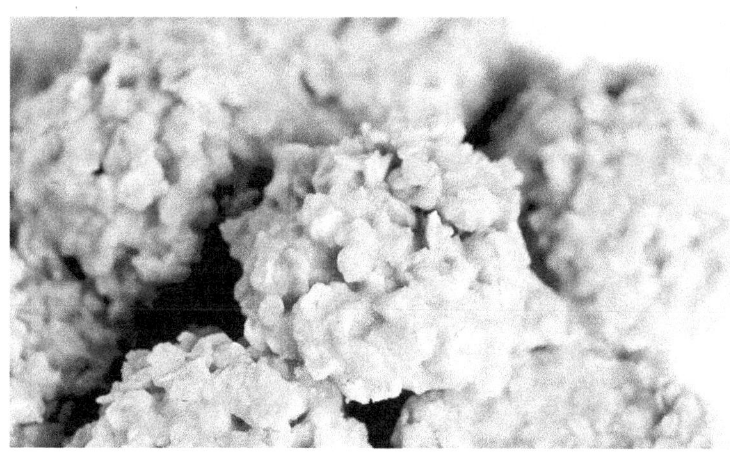

*Preparation time*: 05 minutes | *Cooking time*: 05 minutes | *Servings*: 40

## Ingredients:

- ¾ cup soften butter
- 3 cups white sugar
- ½ teaspoon vanilla extract
- ¾ cup milk
- 4 cups quick-cooking oats
- 1 ½ cups soften peanut butter

## Directions:

Take a saucepan and add butter, sugar, and milk. Heat it over the medium flame. When it starts boiling cook it for one minute. Now remove it from the stove and add peanut butter, vanilla extract, and oats in it. Mix all the ingredients until they merged and batter starts to cool down. Set the better in the tray in the form of cookies and leave it to cool down.

**Nutrition:** Fats 7.5g, Calories 152, Carbohydrates 19.4g, Protein 3.2g, Cholesterol 8mg

# Apple Pie

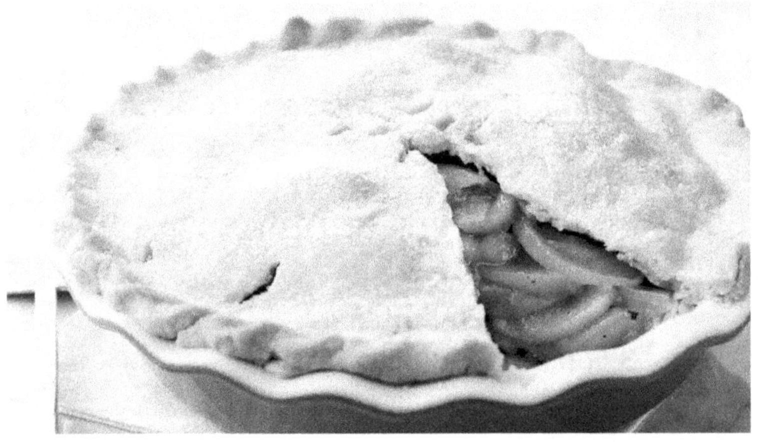

*Preparation time:* *30 minutes |* ***Cooking time****: 01 hour |* ***Servings****: 8*

**Ingredients:**

- 7 cups peeled and sliced apples
- ½ cup granulated sugar
- 3 tablespoons flour
- ½ teaspoon ground cinnamon
- 1 tablespoon lemon juice
- 1/8 teaspoon nutmeg
- 1 double-crust pie pastry

- 1 teaspoon coarse sugar
- 1 beaten egg white

## Directions:

In a bowl mix all the ingredients leaving the last three from the list. Take the baking plate and set the double-crust pie pastry in a proper way. Add prepared apple mixture in it. After filling it, cover it from the remaining dough. Seal its edges properly and remove the excess dough. Make small cuts and brush beaten egg white on its top and sprinkle sugar. Bake it in the 425F preheated oven for 15 minutes and after 15 minutes set the temperature at 375F and bake for 40 minutes more.

**Nutrition:** Fats 12g, Calories 318, Carbohydrates 49g, Protein 3g, Fiber 3g, Sugar 22g

# Choco & Fruit Mousse

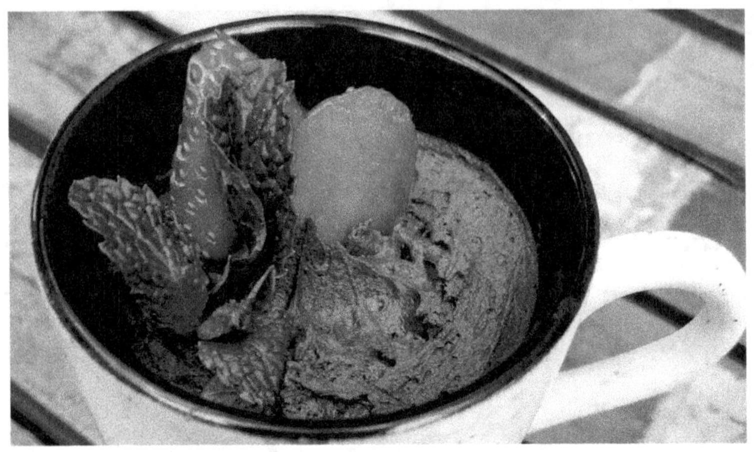

*Preparation time*:  5 minutes / *Chilling time*:  5 minutes / *Servings*: 1

## Ingredients:

- 1 peeled banana
- 1 cup low-fat milk
- 1 tablespoon cocoa powder
- 1 tablespoon maple syrup
- 1 tablespoon chia seeds

## Directions:

Take a blender and put banana, milk, cocoa powder, chia seeds, and maple syrup and blend it well. Blend it for almost one minute if you have a high power blender. And if you are using low power blender blend it for around 2 minutes. Now pour it in the glass and keep it in the refrigerator for just 5 minutes. If you have to serve it immediately then add ice cubes in it.

**Nutrition:** Fats 5g, Calories 314, Carbohydrates 68g, Protein 6g, Sugar 32g, Fiber 11g

# Chocolate Smoothie

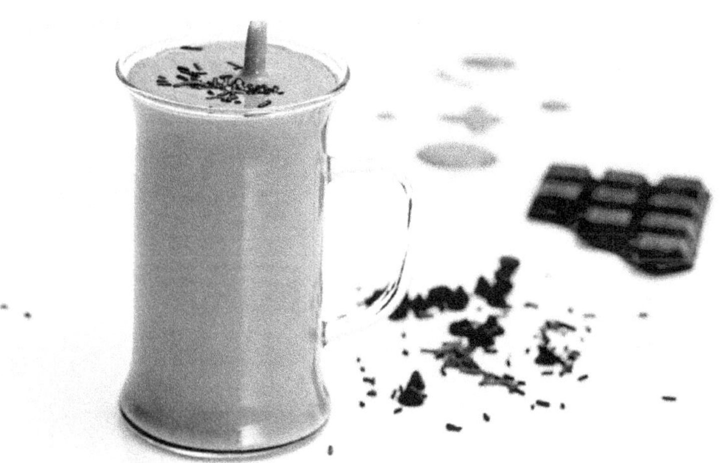

*Preparation time*:  *15 minutes* | ***Chilling time***:  *60 minutes* | ***Servings***: *6*

## Ingredients:

- 1 tablespoon sugar
- 2 cups cream
- 5 egg yolks
- 1 tablespoon vanilla extract
- 5 egg whites
- 4 oz. chocolate chunks
- 1 tablespoon instant coffee
- 1 cup fruit sliced fruit of your choice

**Directions:**

Add cream in a bowl and whip it perfectly. Now add sugar and vanilla extract and blend it well. Melt the chocolate in a boiler. Take a bowl and add egg yolks in it one by one. Mix it well and leave it for 5 minutes. Take another bowl and stir egg whites and add them in the chocolate mixture. Now take a cup and add fruits in its base (fruits can be kiwis, banana, litchis, strawberry, litchis, and so on). Add chocolate mousse and cream mixture in the cup in the form of layers. Refrigerate it for at least 60 minutes and then serve it.

**Nutrition:** Fats 38g, Calories 481, Carbohydrates 28g, Protein 8g

# Grilled Cheese Bites

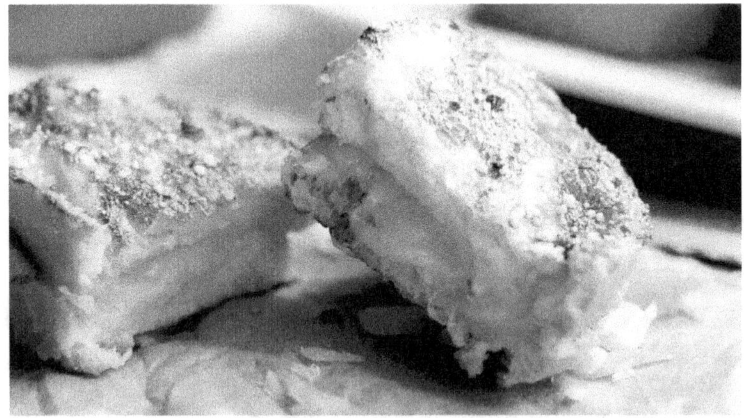

***Preparation time:*** *10 minutes I* ***Cooking time:*** *10 minutes I* ***Servings****: 6*

## Ingredients:

- 1 cup grated cheese
- 1 ounce prepared pizza dough
- 1½ tablespoons garlic powder
- 1 tablespoon olive oil

## Directions:

Preheat the oven at the 400 degrees F temperature. Roll the pizza dough till the ¼ inch thickness. Make the 24 circles with the help of a jar. Put the small amount of grated cheese on the 12 dough circles and sprinkle garlic powder on it. Now place the plain dough rounds on the rounds with cheese and close it from all sides by pressing it gently. With a brush drizzle, olive oil on each prepared dough bites and place it in the baking tray. Bake it in the preheated oven for around 10 minutes.

**Nutrition:** Fats 35g, Calories 457, Carbohydrates 31g, Protein 6g

# Chopped Chickpea Salad

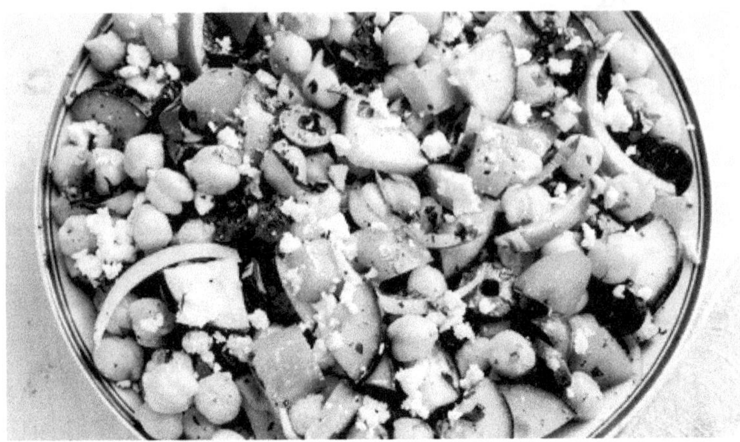

***Preparation time****: 10 minutes | **Chilling time***: 60 minutes | ***Servings***: 4

## Ingredients:

- 1 cup rinsed and drained chickpeas
- 3 chopped bell peppers
- 1 cup diced tomatoes
- 1 sliced cut cucumber
- ¼ cup cubed cut onion
- 1 cup shredded cheese
- 1/3 cup sliced olives
- 1 crushed garlic cloves
- ½ teaspoon crushed salt and pepper
- 1 teaspoon dried oregano
- 2 tablespoons lemon juice
- 2 tablespoons olive oils

## Directions:

Take a bowl and add olive oil, garlic, oregano, salt, pepper and lemon juice in it, mix it well and set aside. Take another bowl, add all the remaining ingredients in it, and combine them well. In the second bowl add the dressing mixture and whisk it well. Place it in the refrigerator for around one hour. After an hour it is ready to serve.

**Nutrition:** Fats 12.3g, Calories 279, Carbohydrates 33.5g, Protein 12.5g, Sugar 12.4g

# Frozen Berry Yogurt

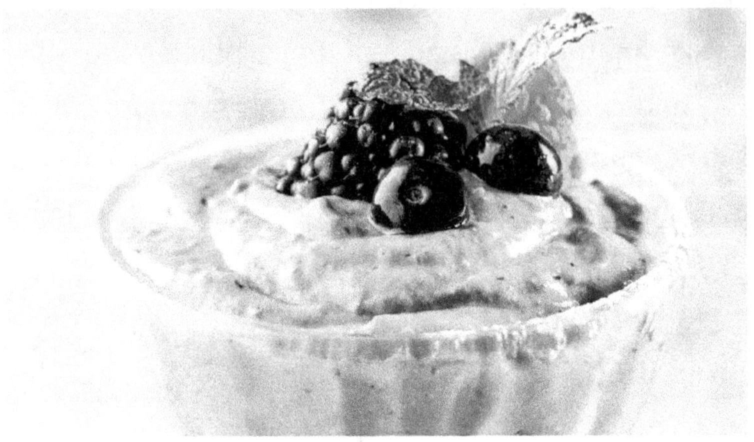

***Preparation time***: *5 minutes* I ***Chilling time***: *3 hours* I ***Servings***: *4*

## Ingredients:

- ½ cup plain yogurt
- 2 cups frozen berries
- 1 teaspoon vanilla essence (optional)
- 2 tablespoons honey

## Directions:

Take a food processor and add all the ingredients. Blend it for 2 minutes or until the ingredients transform in a creamy mixture. Pour it in the ice cream container and put it in the refrigerator for at least 3 hours. Now put it in the serving dish with the help of scoop.

**Nutrition:** Fats 1.2g, Calories 93, Carbohydrates 20.8g, Protein 1.6g, Sugar 17.4g, Cholesterol 4mg

# Choco Bombs

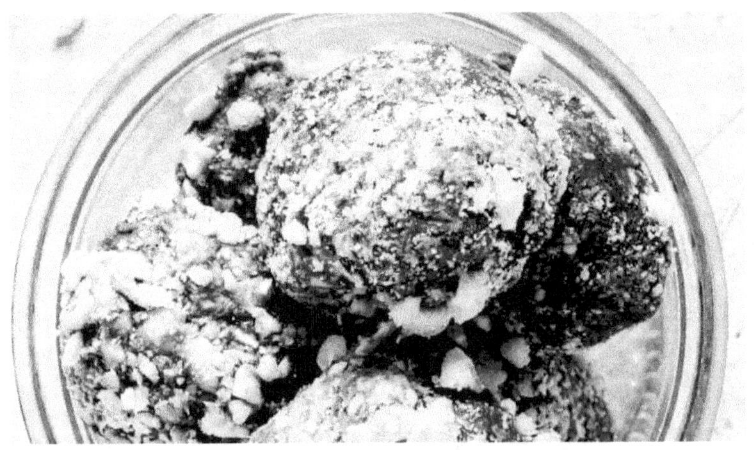

***Preparation time****: 20 minutes I **Chilling time***: *1 hour I **Servings***: *24*

## Ingredients:

- ½ cup white sugar
- 2 tablespoons cocoa powder
- ½ cup margarine
- 2 tablespoons cold coffee
- ½ cup butter
- 1 teaspoon vanilla extract
- 1 ½ cups rolled oats
- ½ cup brown sugar

## Directions:

Take a bowl and whisk the margarine and sugar. Add remaining ingredients except the brown sugar, in it and mix it well until all the ingredients merged well. Take the prepared mixture and make small balls. Sprinkle the brown sugar on these balls and put it in the refrigerator for an hour.

**Nutrition:** Fats 4.1g, Calories 86, Carbohydrates 12.1g, Protein 0.8g.

# Chocolate Chip Muffins

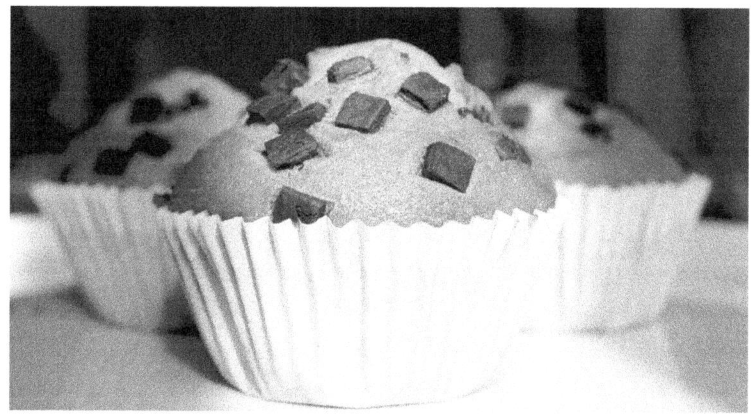

*Preparation time:  15 minutes | **Cooking time**: 30 minutes | **Servings**: 12*

## Ingredients:

- ½ cup melted butter
- 2 eggs

- 2 teaspoons baking powder
- 1 cup crushed sugar
- ½ teaspoon salt
- 2 teaspoons baking soda
- ½ cup milk
- 1 cup chocolate chips
- 2 cups flour
- 1 teaspoon vanilla extract

**Directions:**

Prepare muffin tins with greased liner. Take a bowl and add butter and sugar in it and blend it well. Add the remaining items in the bowl one by one and stir them well. Now pour the prepared batter equally in the muffin cups. Put it in the preheated oven at the 425 degrees F. Bake the muffins for around 25 to 30 minutes or until a toothpick comes out clean when inserted in the middle of a muffin. Transfer them on the serving plate and serve them.

**Nutrition:** Fats 8g, Calories 313, Carbohydrates 41g, Protein 4g, Fiber 1g, Cholesterol 49mg

# Cinnamon cupcake

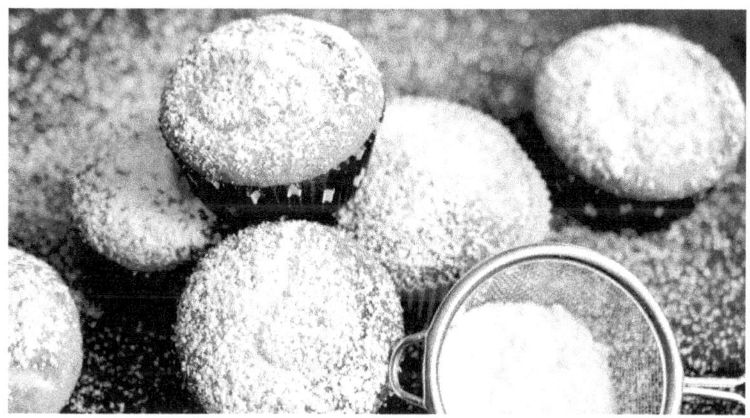

***Preparation time****: 15 minutes | **Cooking time**: 30 minutes | **Servings**: 6*

## Ingredients:

- ½ cup melted butter
- 2 eggs
- ½ cup flour
- 1 cup crushed sugar
- 1 tablespoon cinnamon powder
- 1 teaspoon vanilla extract
- 1 pinch cocoa powder
- 2 teaspoon icing sugar

## Directions:

Prepare muffin tins with greased liner. Preheat the oven at the 350F temperature. Add butter and sugar in a bowl and mix it well. Now add remaining ingredients in it and mix them well until all the ingredients merged well. Put the batter in the prepared muffin try equally and bake it for 20 minutes. Before serving sprinkle icing sugar on it.

**Nutrition:** Fats 19.8g, Calories 436, Carbohydrates 63.9g, Protein 3g, Fiber 1.3, Sugar 49.8g, Cholesterol 34mg.

# Mixed Fruit Trifle

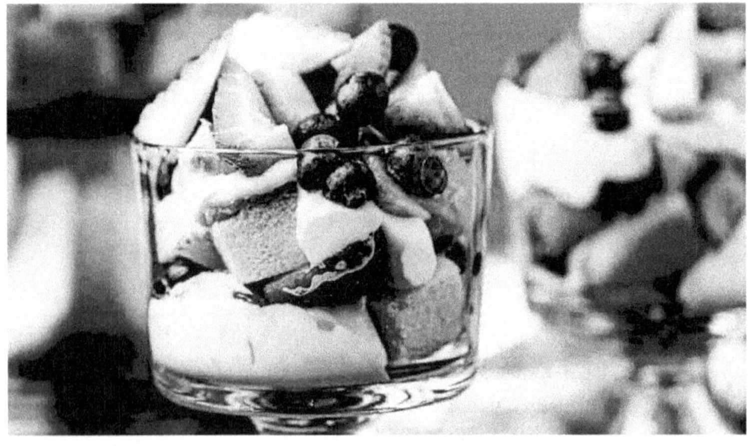

*Preparation time*:  15 *minutes* I ***Chilling time***: 30 *minutes* I **Servings**: 4

## Ingredients:

- 1 marble cake
- 2 cups milk
- 1 cup banana pudding
- ½ teaspoon maple syrup
- 2 cups whipped cream

- 1 bowl frozen mixed fruits

**Directions:**

Take a bowl and beat the cream and sugar. Cut the cake in a small diced form. Take a serving bowl and place the cake pieces in its bottom. Add pudding, prepared cream, and fruits in the form of layers. Put it in the refrigerator for 30 minutes for chilling.

**Nutrition:** Fats 33g, Calories 258, Carbohydrates 55g, Protein 9g, Sugar 27g, Cholesterol 60mg.

## Carrot Cake Bliss Balls

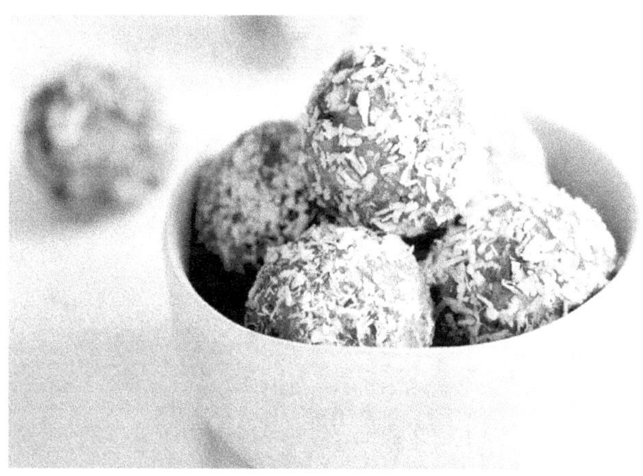

*Preparation time:* *10 minutes I **Chilling time**: 30 minutes I **Servings**: 6*

**Ingredients:**

- 1 cup toasted rolled oats
- ½ cup toasted sunflower seeds
- 6 pitted dates
- ½ cup grated carrots
- 1½ tablespoons cinnamon powder
- 2 teaspoon icing sugar
- 1 pinch cocoa powder
- ½ cup shriveled coconut for coating

**Directions:**

Add all the ingredients in the blender and blend it for around 3 minutes or until all the ingredients are finely chopped and merged well. Take a small amount of batter in your hand and make a ball. Coat it with desiccated coconut. Store the balls in the refrigerator for chilling for around 30 minutes.

**Nutrition:** Fats 2.6g, Calories 87, Carbohydrates 15g, Protein 1.8g, Fiber 2.2, Sugar 8.4g.

# Chapter 12
## 21day Meal Plan

Weight gain and obesity are the growing problems that people are facing nowadays. The main reason behind the issue is inactivity and busy schedule, due to which it is hard to streamline the proper food intake. Moreover, because of undue pressure the intake of junk and unhealthy food are getting higher and that turns everyone's life into an unhealthy one. As the weight gain brings multiple of other health complications together like blood pressure, obesity, blood sugar, anxiety, inflammation and many other issues, to deal with these problems many people adopt different ways of dieting, meal plans, fasting tips and workouts. Some are effective, but everything is not for everyone.

Almost everyone has a different body structure and hormones balance, due to every dieting method, it may not give the same results to everyone. Besides all, intermittent fasting is one of the best and popular way to overcome the excessive weight with the healthy way of fasting and eating. Indeed, in this way of losing weight, a person usually breaks out the day into fasting and eating window that provide opportunity to fast between the meals and boost the overall metabolic function.

The body needs energy to perform the functions properly and without the supply of energy in shape of food intake, body switch towards the stored body fats. It starts cutting down the fats into energy and body utilizing that energy to perform the different tasks, when a person is on fasting condition. Some consultant refers that fasting with the workout gives more effective results in less time, and if a person adds the weight training with the fasting, it will definitely boost the metabolism and protect the muscle mass to reduce. Intermittent fasting is the way that almost suits to everyone.

### What is mean by meal plan?

Meal plans are most effective and beneficial way to limit the quality food intake with the fasting and eating windows. It is highly recommended that the person should follow the proper meal plans that suits the body requirement.

### What about 21-day meal plan?

Eating without thinking may give adverse effect to the health in shape of weight gain. 21-day meat plan is an advanced meal plan that helps to restrict the food options into a specific one. A person who is following the plan has to eat only the listed product that do not need to count the calories before eating, and sometimes for someone even does not need to have a high intensity workout session. In the list of meal plan certain products that are added includes eggs, lean meat, veggies, lemon, lime, limited spices and many other items. Finally, a person has to switch the items each day.

If a person follows the 21-day meal plan with the intermittent fasting method the results will be shown quickly, as it does not only boosts the metabolism but it also helps to keep the stamina and energy level up to the mark.

### Things to list down in 21-day meal plan

In 21-day meal plan person has to include only the restricted items that are defined with the low carbs and calorie food items, but they are able to provide a high amount of energy so the body can survive and act confidently. Here is some food that can be included in 21-day meal plan:

- Low carbs or whole food items
- Low fat dairy products
- Lean meat, fish or eggs
- Non-starchy vegetables
- Brown rice or quinoa
- Legume based pasta
- Almond, walnuts and other nuts those are high in fiber
- Unsweetened or unsalted rice cake
- Almond or peanut butter
- Cottage cheese
- Greek yogurt

While making the 21-day meal plan the most important thing that has to be considered is use the minimum amount of salt or spices, since high salted or spices in the food act as the water retention in the body and can be a source to store the glucose in the body.

### How 21-day meal plan works?

21-day meal plan can be a part of the intermittent fasting and followed in the eating window parallel to the fasting one; it includes the food items that are low in calorie and carbs that make your stomach full for a longer time and helps to avoid the hunger in fasting time. With the appropriate meal and following this plan, it is easy to keep up the body's energy level and the overall mood is improved. A person does not need to count the calories with following the 21-day meal plan because it is already a set form of food items.

By consuming the low-calorie or low carbs food the amount of glucose is not able to store in the body and to boost the metabolism. By increasing the metabolism stored fats and start turning into the energy, the body utilizes that energy into workouts and performs other activities. Eating less calories can keep the fiber and nutrients requirement complete and could switch the habits towards the healthy one. Everyone can have a different meal plan as per the requirement and after consulting the health consultant.

### *Is the 21-day meal plan being effective or not?*

21-day meal plan consist of the list of healthy food items, that are including the whole food, vegetables and non-starchy and salted product. A person can experience an effective weight loss by following the list of some specific food items included in daily meals for almost 21 days consecutively. This plan has a significant impact on the overall health. Consultants recommend that with this meal plan a person should have to consume more water and avoid the consumption of sugar. It boosts the metabolism function that starts breaking down the stored body fats into energy.

By following this plan with the intermittent fasting, it doubles the benefits and is an appropriate choice for both the men and women. This is remarkable for losing the weight in short time frame with the exclusive benefits. There is no need to follow any kind of intense workouts or trainings with such eating habits. A person can have a lean muscle mass with strength and stamina.

### *Benefits of 21-day meal plan*

21-day plan getting popular because it has multiple of health benefits. Some of them are as following:

### *Help to lose weight*

The purpose to promote the weight loss by controlling the consumption of sugary and salted products. As per the studies, it is significant that by cutting down the consumption of sugary products and salted one it is easy to reduce the weight, as well as to promote the consumption of good fats, fibers and proteins in overall diet.

## Healthy eating habits

By fixing the nutritional requirement and focusing more on the fiber and proteins intake, this method leads to a good and healthy eating habits. People who are supposed to follow the diet plan are consciously avoiding the junk, packed and processed food, as well as following the way to cook the healthy and homemade food that are good for the weight loss.

## Give portion control encouragement

Portion control and measuring the portion is an effective way to limit the calorie intake and helps to avoid the overeating, which may lead to weight loss. Usually the cups and spoons are used to have a proper and exact measurement of the portion that a person required to consume in one time as a meal.

## Indulge exercise in the plan

In 21-day meal plan it is suggested to add the exercise or activity of almost 30 minutes. This is effective and keeps the muscles active and gives them strength, because losing or maintaining weight have a significant importance of the exercise and physical activity into the life. So, it is recommended to follow the exercise for almost 30 minutes daily or four days in a week with the meal plans.

# Chapter 13
## Faqs

***What is intermittent fasting?***

Intermittent fasting is an advanced and effective way to make arrangements of having meals and fasting. People follow a proper meal plan window in which they are concerned to have a proper nutritional food and cut down them into segments between eating and fasting. That is all to get the effective benefits to lose weight and follow the healthy lifestyle. People follow different intermitted fasting methods that depends on the requirement and as per their ease. Due to its remarkable benefits, this way of losing weight is getting popular among people around the world.

***Is intermitting fasting effective for weight lose?***

Yes, this is true. Intermittent fasting is an effective and result oriented way to lose weight, especially for people who are living with the obesity and getting sick of the extra fats and want to have a fit and healthy lifestyle. In this, a person can just divide the meals into portions and have them with fasting intervals. This process improves the metabolism and utilizes the store energy to fuel up the body in fasting time.

### What kind of benefits a person can get it from fasting?

Intermittent fasting is no doubt an effective and popular way to be active, fit and to lose weight. It is more recognizable than any other dieting method. Fasting is just not effective to lose weight but is also good for the health improvement, as it helps to improve the blood circulation, metabolism function and reduces the chances of diabetes in the people having obesity. With the fasting inflammation they can be controlled and reduced the chances of heart issue and high blood pressure. Most importantly, fasting improves the hormonal function and improves insulin level in the body.

### Is it safe to do exercise while fasting?

Some people think that exercise with fasting may cause issues and is not appropriate, but in reality, it is really good and effective. Having workout session with fasting not only improves the functions but it also helps to get results in minimum time. So, with exercise a person can build stamina and achieve muscle strength as well.

### What is an ideal fasting ratio?

There are multiple methods designed by the health consultant for fasting and a person can choose one that suits best, as well as it can be selected with the expert opinion. Usually, the most common and ideal intermittent fasting method is 16:8 that is followed by people who want to lose weight. It means that a person has an 8-hour-eating window in a day with 16 hours fasting. A person can modify and alter the fasting hours as per the body's demand.

### *Which time is best for workout?*

People set their priorities according to the body requirement and the results they are targeting to achieve. Usually, the best time or the workout is an hour or two before you have a plan to break your fast; in this time, you can have a full advantage and benefit of exercise. The longer you put the gap and wait between workout and having a meal, the more you will be able to get the benefits.

How to spend day with intermittent fasting?

While following the intermittent fasting it is necessary to follow the proper plan and schedule to spend your whole day. So, adjust the workout timing in between the meal window and, if you follow the morning workout session, then do it before two hours of having a meal to break your fast. If you just skip to have morning training session, then it does not matter because you can adjust it in between your day. However, remember that to get the great results, you should follow the fasting plan at least for a month or long.

### *Is intermittent fasting being safe?*

Intermittent fasting is a safe and result oriented way to lose weight and follow the best outcomes to lose weight. It follows a process in which people just cut down the meal intake that leads calorie deduction without the calorie count. With fasting body functions are improved like metabolism, insulin sensitivity and inflammation that gives multiple health benefits, but those who are facing any serious illness or a chronical disease should follow the fasting method by consulting the health consultant.

### *Can a person build muscle with fasting?*

Usually, with intermittent fasting a person can lose the weight and get lean muscle mass. For the gain it does not have any significant results, but multiple fitness trainers suggest different training or high intensity workouts that help to gain muscle mass as well. High level weight training with the protein intake help to reduce the fats and lean muscle, furthermore, weight lifting protects the muscle lose during fasting.

### *What are health benefits of intermittent fasting?*

Most importantly, intermittent fasting helps to reduce the weight and gets a chance to maintain an ideal one, as it is an effective way to have a healthy body and a sound mind. Parallel to this, there are multiple other health benefit a person can enjoy with this, it includes:

- An effective way to lose weight without losing muscle mass.

- It helps to improve insulin level and reduces the inflammation in blood and body.
- Improves the heart health and reduces the risk of heart attack.
- Improves overall strength and stamina and revitalizes the body functions.

## A diabetic can fast or not?

Intermittent fasting helps to improve the insulin sensitivity and maintains the optimal level in the body. According to the health consultants' diabetics can follow the intermittent fasting but it is preferred to consult the doctor before starting, because it directly influences the hormonal level, as well as other functions of the body and may cause the risk of hypoglycemia, this means a condition of low blood sugar level due to limited consumption of the calories and nutrients.

## Why intermittent fasting getting popular?

The simple and schedule eating habits are good for the health and they maintain an optimal healthy weight. However, in today's busy schedule it is hard to follow for almost everyone, but intermitted fasting brings it back into the practice, because it is a different and effective way to control the weight and it leads an active lifestyle. Furthermore, it is getting popular because it brings ease and simplicity in life and now you do not need to count calories or prepare a special meal other than routine.

### Is it safe to have supplements or a person can take them with fasting?

Yes, you can consume the supplements while having the intermittent fasting. But the most important thing that you have to consider is not to follow high calorie supplements with the meals. Try to use them with the workout plans. Although, instead of having supplements it is preferable to consume high protein and whole food into the meal window, for the better results.

### Who should avoid fasting?

Fasting have a significant effect for almost everyone in form of good weight management and health, but not everyone can follow the fasting in same pattern. People with serious health issue have to consult the expert before starting. So, do not follow the intermittent fasting if you are:

- On a medication
- You have diabetes or an issue of low blood sugar level
- You are under weight
- Have low blood pressure issue
- Suffering from any chronical disease
- A woman who is trying to conceive
- Pregnant and breast-feeding woman
- A person who has any digestive problem

### *What kind of liquids are allowed in fasting?*

While following the fasting you should have to add low calorie drinks into your routine. Thus, consume more water and use electrolytes to improve the metabolic process, as well as coffee or tea without sugar or milk can be consumed. A person has to avoid the sugary drinks and carbonated or energy drinks.

### *Will the intermittent fasting slow down metabolism?*

No, that's not true, in fact, intermittent fasting has a good effect on a person's metabolism function, as it not only boosts the metabolism but it also helps to improve the blood circulation. Moreover, it helps to utilize the stored fats as a source of energy that body utilizes during the fasting period and at the time of exercise. Finally, it effectively reduces the weight and helps obesity.

### *Will fasting cause the muscle loss?*

According to the general studies, it is noticed that the intense fasting and high intensity workout may lead to loss of the muscle mass with the weight. To avoid such situation, it is recommended to follow the high intensity weight trainings. Through weight training muscles got the strength and person can improve the stamina; besides, it also prevents the muscle loss and keeps it strong and lean.

### Is intermittent fasting safe for women?

As compared to men, intermittent fasting is not highly recommended for women because it can cause the hormonal changes that leads to certain health complications. According to the studies, it is evident that the fasting effects the menstruation cycle and ovulation process as well. That may cause the problems of infertility and other. So, a woman who is looking to follow intermittent fasting to lose weight, it is recommended to consult the doctor and a health advisor first before starting.

### What are the top tips to follow during intermittent fasting?

Intermittent fasting is no doubt an effective and most popular way to diet and lose weight nowadays. There are some tips that a person should follow while following the method of fasting. Here are the tips:

- Consume excessive water throughout a day to keep body hydrated
- Listen to the body first and break your fast, if you feel the body is exhausted and it needs energy
- Do not miss any meal from the schedule
- Consume low calorie drinks to fuel up the body
- Be consistent with the fasting and you should follow for at least a month or two to get the remarkable changes
- Choose the healthy or whole food during the eating period of your schedule

- Have low-calorie and low card diet to make your stomach feel full and avoid the hunger during the fasting time period.
- If you have any eating disorder and other chronical health problem, then stop doing the fasting and consult the health consultant first.

### Is this being safe for the children as well?

For children, intermittent fasting is not suitable and not recommended to follow because it leads a low nutrients and mineral supply, which can be dangerous for the kids.

### Does a person need to cut more calories with fasting?

No, that's not necessary to cut more calories from the meal window while following the intermittent fasting plans, because during fasting it is necessary to follow a proper count of calorie and, if a person stays on low calorie diet for a long time with fasting, it will turn down the metabolism function.

# Conclusion

People are considering the ways to lose weight effectively but they don't want to compromise the health and they want effective results that sustain for a longer time. Intermittent fasting brings a blessing into the person's life who is dealing with the obesity, or other weight related issue and was not able to find out a solution to get rid of it. In market multiple of weight loss supplements, diet plans and methods are available and they guarantee slim and fit physique. However, every method or product is not useful for everyone; but that is not the case of intermittent fasting, because it is not a medication or a supplement, it is simply a method or a lifestyle changes, in which a person adopts too fast for the certain time in a day and eats limited and healthy food to get the full health benefits.

There are different methods of fasting and eating that anyone can choose the one that suits the body or as per the requirements. In this fasting procedure consultant suggested to keep the body hydrated and consume more water and nonalcoholic or low-calorie drinks to support the metabolism. Fasting has multiple other health benefits as well, such as: it helps to reduce the risk of heart disease, diabetics, treat the inflammation, which are good for people having insomnia issue and other remarkable benefits. According to few researches the intermittent fasting is not as supported for women as men, because it can change the hormonal balances that lead health complication and other fertility issues in females. However, for a safe zone woman can do intermittent fasting, but with a proper consultation.

People who want to find out the benefits and looking to start the intermittent fasting can facilitate with this piece of literature that will help to identify the methods to do fasting, as well as a person can better find out the best option by reviewing the all-pros and cons and other factors that can influence the better outcomes and much more. Furthermore, this book provides a comprehensive detail about intermittent fasting and the way through a person can start it well to get the maximum benefits out of it.

Jennifer.